DATE DUE

NOV 2 8 1997	
JUL 1 4 1998	

BRODART   Cat. No. 23-221

The Cancer Nurse's Perspective: Stress and the Person with Cancer

A musician must make music, an artist must paint, a poet must write, if he is to be ultimately at peace with himself. What a man can be, he must be.

Maslow, Abraham Harold
Motivation and Personality (1954)

This book is dedicated with love to my parents.

Acknowledgements

I am indebted to the Department of Health for their financial support of my doctoral research programme. I was awarded a Department of Health Research Studentship which enabled me to pursue my research full-time and to acquire an educational grounding in research, for a period of three years.

As this work was funded by the Department of Health, the text is covered by Crown Copyright and this must be acknowledged when the work is quoted:

© *Crown Copyright 1991*

I would like to acknowledge the support of my supervisor, Prof Chris Henry.

The Cancer Nurse's Perspective: Stress and the Person with Cancer

by

Elizabeth Jane Hanson

Quay Publishing Limited
Nereus House, New Quay Road
Lancaster, LA1 5SA

British Library Cataloguing in Publication Data
A catalogue record of this book is available from the British Library

© 1994 Hanson, E J

IBN 1 85642 079 5

Contents

Introduction

As a staff nurse working on a general oncology ward, I was frequently made aware, through everyday work on the ward, of the importance of psychological aspects of cancer nursing care. I realised that insufficient emphasis was placed upon how the person with cancer was feeling psychologically on a daily basis. If this aspect was explored, it was not always communicated systematically. As a result, the psychological needs of individuals with cancer were often not cared for soon enough. This then led to an exacerbation of the individuals' problems and increased levels of stress.

I realised that, on first admission to hospital, the person with cancer has not only to cope with a strange environment and people, but also with the additional stress associated with the knowledge or suspicion of a diagnosis of cancer. Through my own experience of cancer nursing, it became increasingly obvious that the cancer nurse needs to play a fundamental part in helping persons with cancer overcome their stress as much as possible, not only on admission, but throughout the course of their stay in hospital.

This provided the impetus for the current study. I aimed to explore the views of cancer nurses regarding stress in persons with cancer, in order to make a further contribution to the knowledge of stress applied to individuals with cancer, and also to explore the ways in which cancer nurses assess stress in persons with cancer. I chose cancer nurses as the focus of the study due to my previous cancer nursing experience. I am of the opinion that cancer nurses, in their everyday work experiences, have the most contact with individuals with cancer. In addition, due to the nurses' role as patient advocate, they have a special helping relationship. As a result, it can be acknowledged that cancer nurses are likely to possess a rich working knowledge of stress and persons with cancer.

I carried out a thorough literature review of psychological theories of stress and related psychological concepts, in order to give a firm theoretical underpinning for the subsequent study. The research methods chosen were those that would most closely match the aims of the study. The results were then fed back directly to the theory to provide the data for a critical discussion of the views of cancer nurses in relation to stress as applied to persons with cancer. This then allowed a theoretical framework to be put forward, to act as an appropriate educational foundation for nurses in relation to their psychosocial care of individuals with cancer.

Aims of the study

1 To undertake a theoretical study of the concept of stress applied to person with cancer as perceived by cancer nurses.

2 To study the view of qualified members of nursing staff concerning the concept of stress amongst individuals with cancer.

3 To observe the nursing admission assessment of persons with cancer, in order to explore the effects of the cancer nurse upon the person with cancer in relation to information regarding their perceived stress.

4 To identify common areas of concern, as perceived by cancer nurses, which may lead to appraisals of stress amongst persons with cancer.

5 To develop an appropriate knowledge base for cancer nurses regarding the nursing care of persons with cancer.

A phenomenological approach

A broad phenomenological approach was adopted because its philosophy closely links to the overall perspective of Lazarus' transactional model of stress (1966). Phenomenology bases its roots in the history of philosophy in the late nineteenth century as a clear move away from the popular approach of positivism, with its emphasis upon seeking facts and causes of social phenomenon. Its inspiration was derived from philosophers such as Hesserl, Spiegelberg and Giorgi, who reacted against the natural sciences and their emphasis upon objectifying human behaviour. Instead, they sought to explain the phenomenon of the human being, as they argued that people cannot be controlled in the same manner that natural phenomena can be controlled. Herein lies the essential difference between the two perspectives of phenomenology and positivism. The concept of the person as opposed to the concept of a thing, is the main strand of phenomenology as a philosophy and an approach (Henry, 1987).

The medical model encompasses the tenets of a positivistic approach because it reduces the patient to the lowest common denominator, i.e. cells and atoms. This is often referred to as biological reductionism, which allows very little room for the expression of higher order concepts, such as thoughts, feelings and emotions. The medical model reflects the dominant influence upon nursing since the nineteenth century. The chief means for nursing to gain respectability and professional status was to describe nursing as being mainly concerned with carrying out medical directives. The traditional image of the nurse is one of subservience to medical colleagues. As a result, nursing has remained in the shadow of medicine and the philosophy of biomedicine has strongly influenced the development of both basic and post-basic courses in nurse education (Kendrick, 1991; Witts, 1991). This argument relates directly to the criticism directed at the cancer nurse and the failure to adopt an active psychological support role.

The focus of the phenomenological approach is understanding human behaviour from the agent's perspective. The individual's experience in everyday life events is a central theme, the premise being that there is value in exploring the meaning of any event or experience that affects human beings. People act toward people and things on the basis of the meaning these things have for them, i.e. meaning determines action. People attach meanings to situations, other things and themselves though a process of interpretation. They are constantly interpreting and defining things as they move through different situations. This reflects my study, as the main aim is to gain a deeper understanding of the concept of stress amongst individuals with cancer as perceived by individual nurses. The key words in phenomenology are 'meaning' and 'understanding'; the notion that there is value in exploring the meaning of any event or experience that affects human beings.

Thus, for this research project, it can be seen that a phenomenological approach and the use of qualitative research methods were appropriate. My main aim was to study the complex meaning of stress of individuals with cancer, as perceived by cancer nurses, through the use of explanations surrounding meaning, interpretation and understanding.

1 Psychological theories of stress

What follows is a critical review of the main psychological theories of stress, in order to provide an appropriate foundation for the subsequent exploration of the views of cancer nurses regarding stress in relation to persons with cancer.

Selye's response-based model of stress

Selye's approach (1957) is largely a medical model, being firmly based in physiology. He proposed that it is necessary to look for a particular pattern of responses, which can be taken as evidence that a person is stressed. Thus, the occurrence of a response represents the occurrence of stress, which may act as a stimulus for producing further responses. Selye's main view of stress is the non-specificity and universality of the physiological response of the body to any demand made upon it: the 'general adaptation syndrome' (GAS). If the stress continues, resources dwindle, collapse and, finally, disease states occur as the costs of defence.

Selye's response model is a restrictive approach to the study of stress. It has since been argued that Selye overstates the concept of non-specificity because specificity is evident. For example, heart rates and respiratory rates differ from one person to another. Selye's physiological-oriented model fails to reveal an interaction between physiological and psychological factors. Clearly, both factors are involved, but as Lazarus (1966) states, the most important factor to consider is the individual's perception of the situation as stressful or not. Selye's model loses sight of the individual because it is a general theory which focuses on **'scientific generality'**.

For the purposes of the study, Selye's response model is not the most appropriate perspective for the following reasons. First, it clearly makes use of a medical model and, second, there is a lack of interactive aspects and concern for the individual's perceptions of stress.

Stimulus-based model of stress

A stimulus approach to stress is based on a medical/engineering model and considers which external stressors in the environment lead to the stress response. Stress occurs whenever the demand for adaptation made on an organism departs from a moderate level. Low levels of demand on an individual can be as stressful as high levels of demand. Most organisms, including man, have evolved to produce optimum adaptive performance under conditions of moderate demand (Cox, 1978).

A stimulus approach to stress is concerned with trying to identify situations which can be reliably described as stressful to man. Holmes and Rahe (1967) attempted to quantify the degree of stress associated with life events. They constructed a scale of 43 life events. The authors found that death of a spouse was consistently rated highest and this was given a value of 100. All other events were given proportional values based on this. The authors claimed to have revealed that people in the United States, Western Europe and Japan tend to rate life events in almost exactly the same pattern.

The main criticism of a stimulus-based model, similar to that of a response-based model, is that it fails to take into account the individual and his/her personal perception of a situation. As a result, it does not address individual differences with regard to a particular situation. Lazarus (1981) criticises both these conventional approaches to stress, as they view the person and environment as separate entities. They fail to see the importance of the person and his/her environment being examined in relation to one another.

The transactional model of stress

The transactional model of stress and coping has been selected as the theoretical framework for this study, because of the central importance of the individual's role in perceiving stress. Lazarus (1966) states that stress occurs when there are demands on the person which tax or exceed his/her adjustive resources. He continues by explaining that stress is **not** simply 'out there' in the environment, although it may originate there. Stress depends not only on the external conditions (environment/situation factors), but also on the vulnerabilities of the individual and the adequacy of his/her system of defences (personality factors). Thus, he argues that we cannot be ready for a general theory, until we have a satisfactory analysis of psychological stress at the level of the person. Lazarus attempts to do this.

The concept of the uniqueness of the person described in the transactional model is highly relevant to the world of nursing and the use of the nursing process, which emphasises treating patients as individuals, each with their respective needs. The transactional model of stress also begins to explore the complex role of cognition, which is a key concept relating directly to stress and coping. Thus, how the person perceives a situation influences whether or not he/she will experience stress and, if so, how he/she will subsequently deal with it. This closely links to the phenomenological approach which focuses upon the meaning of an event for the individual concerned.

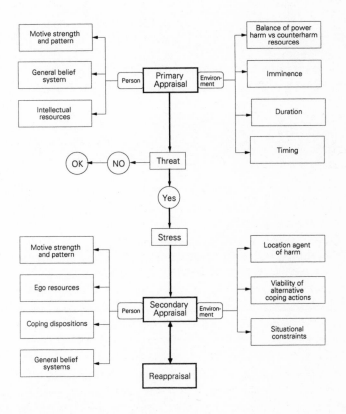

Figure 1.1: Diagrammatic representations of Lazarus' transactional model of stress and coping (1966)

Within the transactional model of stress, the individual is viewed positively as playing an active part in influencing his/her environment as opposed to a passive role. The emphasis upon the active role of the individual reflects the current move within nursing philosophy towards self care and personal responsibility for health, away from the traditional medical view of the patient as a passive being (see Fig. 1.1).

Threat and appraisal

The concept of threat is at the centre of Lazarus' work on stress. He defines threat as occurring when an individual anticipates confrontation with a harmful condition. He carefully points out that the exact conditions that produce threat will vary according to the individual. Lazarus argues that the concept of threat is closely linked to the cognitive process of **appraisal**. Appraisal consists of how a person construes a situation, i.e. whether it is viewed as beneficial, benign or harmful. In other words, for threat to occur, an evaluation must be made of the situation to the effect that harm is signified. Lazarus admits that appraisal is a cognitive process of considerable complexity and abstractness. For example, appraisal is often taken to be a conscious, rational and deliberate process. However, threat appraisal can arise without the person concerned clearly knowing the values and goals that are evaluated as endangered.

Lazarus attempts to examine appraisal in order to gain a deeper insight into psychological stress. He refers to primary appraisal as the cognitive process of evaluating the significance of an encounter for one's well-being, i.e. 'Am I OK or am I in trouble?' Lazarus first studies factors in the environment that determine threat appraisal. Although it may appear to the reader that Lazarus' approach is, in effect, similar to a traditional stimulus-response approach as he studies factors in the environment, it does differ radically as he emphasises the interaction between the individual and environment. Lazarus only separates the two for the purpose of examining these main concepts. Lazarus later clarifies this himself, as he emphasises the difference in approach from the stimulus approach, because there are great individual variations in the extent to which events are appraised as being stressful. Thus, he carefully states that he is **not** concerned with actual 'stressful' events or the normative rank of ordering stressful events, reflective of a stimulus-based model of stress.

Stress situation (environment) factors

- The relative balance of power between the harm-producing stimulus to be confronted and the counter-harm resources of the individual and environment. The more powerful the anticipated event to produce harm in relation to the individual's resources, the greater the likelihood of threat appraisal. On the other hand, the more powerful the resources for mastering the harmful confrontation, the less likely is the threat appraisal. An example of counter-harm resources is the support an individual may receive from significant others, friends and support agencies.

- The imminence of the confrontation in the environment. If the advent of harm is distant, the degree of threat is likely to be low.

- The ambiguity of stimulus cues concerning the harm. This usually intensifies threat because it limits the individual's sense of control or increases his/her sense of helplessness with respect to the danger. Lazarus states that ambiguity allows for idiosyncratic interpretations of situations, based on an individual's psychological structure. (See p63 for Seligman's work (1975) and also p29 regarding the uncertainty of cancer.)

- The duration, i.e. how long a stressful event persists. Lazarus argues that this forms a major consideration in disease. He notes, however, that the damaging effects of a chronic stressor can be mediated through coping and reappraisal.

- The timing of stressful events in relation to the life cycle. Thus, whether or not the life events are expectable. If an event is too early, one is deprived of the support of compatible peers and it often deprives the person of a chance to prepare for a new role. However, if an event is too late, the individual is deprived of the full sense of pride and satisfaction which would accompany the event had it been on time.

Stress personality factors

- The motivational characteristics of the individual. Lazarus argues that people will react with stress in a similar way to a given situation only when they share certain motives that are threatened. Yet, motives tend to vary among different individuals, thus, what is perceived as threatening will also vary.

- An individual's general belief system regarding the environment and one's capacity to control it. General beliefs refer to a total outlook that has no connection with the specific environment, except through broad generalisation. Thus, it is a disposition rather than a specific evaluation. For example, the environment may be seen as powerful, unmanageable or readily subject to control. The tendency to appraise threat readily may itself be regarded as a personality trait. For example, individuals with a disposition towards anxiety may react with threat appraisals to situations that are not explicitly threatening.

- An individual's intellectual resources, i.e. a person's knowledge, may help to determine an inference that a cue signifies harm. If an individual has low levels of intellectual competence they may be oblivious of certain cues, thus limiting their counter-harm resources. This may well lead to the individual being increasingly vulnerable to threats. However, a person with many intellectual resources may, on some occasions, make increased threat appraisals, as their relevant knowledge of a situation may lead to increased scepticism. For example, a nurse diagnosed with metastatic breast cancer, who has full knowledge of the long-term prognosis, may be extremely dubious of a doctor's reassurances that she will be 'cured'.

To summarise, primary appraisal consists of evaluating a situation as threatening or non-threatening. There are two key variables which affect the appraisal. First, are factors in the environment: the balance of power between harm and counter-harm resources, the imminence of the confrontation, the ambiguity of the stimulus cues concerning harm and the duration and timing of stressful events. Second, are the factors within an individual's psychological structure: the motive strength and pattern, general belief systems regarding transactions with the environment and intellectual resources. Although Lazarus examines the main factors influencing an individual's perceptions of stress, it is highly likely, given the complex nature of stress, that a possible multitude of factors remain unexplored.

Secondary appraisal

If primary appraisal begins to answer the question 'How much am I in danger (if any) from a situation?', then secondary appraisal begins to answer the more complex question of 'To what extent will any particular action relieve the danger?' Thus, secondary appraisal involves the process of coping. Lazarus (1966) defines coping as what an individual does to handle stressful demands. It is a form of problem solving in which the stakes are an individual's wellbeing. Often, the individual is not fully clear about what to do. Lazarus takes care to note that this cognitive process is often nearly instantaneous and it is commonly a symbolic process. However, he attempts to describe in detail the key factors involved in the concept of appraisal.

The concept of threat is also central to the process of secondary appraisal. In particular, the **degree** of threat is directly linked with coping. Lazarus states that the more adaptive and reality-oriented forms of coping are most likely when threat is comparatively mild. Likewise, under severe threat more repressive and pathological forms of coping are the norm. (See p13 on coping and the work of Weisman (1979), regarding extreme forms of coping by persons with cancer.)

The motivating properties of threat are also linked with coping. That is, the more important the endangered goal, the more extreme will be the coping measures activated to prevent the harm. (For the person with cancer whose life is threatened, it is likely that more extreme forms of coping will be present. See p13 on coping.) Similar to his description of primary appraisal, Lazarus (1966) studies factors in the environment and factors within an individual's psychological structure to understand the process of secondary appraisal more fully.

Coping situation (environment) factors

- The location of the agent of harm. That is, unless an agent of harm is identified, direct forms of coping (avoidance or attack) are not possible, because one must be able to avoid or attack something in particular. Thus, ambiguity associated with an inability to locate the threatening agent, involves vagueness regarding what can be done to decrease the danger when danger is appraised. Location of the agent of harm also involves whether it is within the individual, in the form of inadequacies or conflicting motives, or within the environment. If danger is external, the individual often takes active steps to reduce it. However, if it is within the individual, defence is the probable form of coping.

- The viability of alternative coping actions. The person chooses strategies from his/her available repertoire on the basis of the apparent viability of the action. By viability Lazarus means that it must be an action the individual is capable of and successful in to some extent, in order to master the threat. Actions that are not possible, or dangerous, are apt to be rejected.
- The situational constraints. These make an individual's ideal coping strategy unacceptable because it exposes him/her to threat from a different source, e.g. social norms or pressures.

Coping personality factors

- The motivational pattern of an individual. Certain action tendencies activated for coping with the threat may be further threatening, either due to situational constraints, as explained in factors of the environment, or due to internalised social values.
- The resources of an individual. Lazarus explains that certain personality traits are traditionally assumed to reduce vulnerability to threat and facilitate healthy forms of coping. For example, those who possess ego integrity are not as prone to despair as those who lack it.
- Coping dispositions. Lazarus gives defence as an example of coping dispositions. An individual who is said to possess a defensive disposition is described as having a particular personality trait. In this example, the individual is likely to use defensive forms of coping. However, Lazarus is careful to acknowledge that there is both consistency and variability in the use of coping processes. Thus, individuals possessing an organised system of dispositions also actively respond to situational pressures and are capable of appraising the consequences of their actions as they develop and gain experience from transactions with the environment.
- General beliefs regarding the environment and one's resources. For example, if an individual believes the environment is dangerous/overpowering and feels his/her resources are inadequate to cope with it, the individual is likely to appraise threat chronically. The individual is also apt to use flight and avoidance as coping processes, rather than attack. An individual's coping resources also help to provide the basis of coping action.

To summarise, secondary appraisal consists of evaluating an encounter with respect to coping. Two key variable which affect the appraisal are factors in the environment (the location of the agent of harm, the viability of alternative coping action and situational constraints) and factors within an individual's psychological structure (the motive strength and pattern, ego resources, coping dispositions and general beliefs regarding the environment and one's resources). The degree of threat also affects secondary appraisal. It does not belong to the two factors above, but is a complex intervening product of both.

Coping patterns

Lazarus further explores coping reaction patterns and the appraisals that underlie them. He states that there are two general classes of coping: first, there are action tendencies aimed at eliminating/mitigating the anticipated harmful confrontation (i.e. direct action, Lazarus, 1976); second, there are purely cognitive manoeuvres through which appraisal is altered without action, directed at changing the objective situation (i.e. palliation).

Direct-action tendencies

- Actions aimed at strengthening the individual's resources against the anticipated harm (i.e. preparing against harm). These actions take the form of considered and controlled strategy (for strengthening the means available to master the threat). For example, the use of attack (i.e. aggression) constitutes a primitive form of coping and is often used when there is an external threat of some kind. It is important to note that it may occur only as an action tendency, or it may be expressed overtly in behaviour. The effect of such an action is the stress emotion of anger.

- Avoidance is a basic form of coping in humans when threatened by an agent that is overwhelmingly powerful and/or dangerous. The effect of such an action often results in the stress emotion of fear.

- Inaction occurs when the individual is totally resigned that there are no direct ways of preventing harm. The individual often feels hopeless and this can lead to the stress emotion of depression.

These forms of direct action are simplistic. In reality, there are likely to be variations on these universal types, depending on the exact nature of a situation. Lazarus' early work on coping, particularly in relation to ego resources and coping dispositions, reflects a mechanistic approach which is in conflict with his overriding humanistic approach towards stress.

Defensive reappraisals

Lazarus refers to the second class of coping, which involves cognitive manoeuvres, as defensive reappraisals. Threat is reduced in the mind of the individual, but **not** in reality. Lazarus states that defensive reappraisal involves primitive thought processes, because it is a distortion of reality. He acknowledges that defensive reappraisal is only adaptive when it allows the individual to be more comfortable and not to be seriously disrupted in other ongoing activities. Often, it is maladaptive as it prevents the use of cognitive processes that lead to realistic expectations of a situation and to a tolerance of inevitable later events.

There has been much work undertaken on the subject of defence reappraisals within the last twenty years. Lazarus (1976) acknowledges Freud's earlier writings (1924) upon defence mechanisms and he summarises Freud's fundamental examples, i.e. identification, displacement, repression, reaction formation, projection and intellectualisation. Lazarus acknowledges that there are problems with how defences are recognised (e.g. by inconsistencies in statements, contradiction of words and non-verbal clues). The more successful the defence, the less evidence there will be of the stress reaction. Thus, it is sometimes difficult to know exactly when an individual is using a defence mechanism.

Lazarus (1976) criticises the adequacy of these existing categories in describing all the varieties of threat-reducing psychological mechanisms employed by individuals. There may well be certain behaviours that appear to have threat-reducing properties which are difficult to fit into existing traditional categories. However, over the last ten to fifteen years, writers have acknowledged this problem and there has been a vast input of information regarding patterns and styles of coping. Lazarus (1978) criticises those which give emphasis to coping style and disposition and not to coping processes as they actually occur. There are few studies which are descriptive of how the individual actually handles a particular harm.

In his early study of the basic coping-reaction patterns, Lazarus is careful to point out that the stress emotions (i.e. anger, jealousy, fear, anxiety, guilt depression, grief and shame) are **products** of stressful relationships with the environment. Much of the more recent literature on stress emotions wrongly treat them as **precursors** to stress or as being synonymous with stress itself. Lazarus explains that, when a situation is seen as harmful by the individual, it leads to stress emotion(s) which involve complex disturbances. He examines anxiety-reaction patterns in more detail. Anxiety-reaction is anticipatory and consists of something more harmful in the future. It usually involves highly symbolic dangers, e.g. loss of self. The nature of the dangers and potential adjustments is highly ambiguous. The emotion can vary from a vague feeling or apprehension or unease to a severe sense of foreboding. In some instances, anxiety occurs when a previously successful defensive reappraisal breaks down and threat is again reappraised. In other instances, the action tendency for coping with threat itself is judged as placing the individual in some danger, and anxiety results.

In his later work, Lazarus (1978 and 1981) acknowledges that his past discussion of secondary appraisal is incomplete. he emphasises that appraisal consists of a continuously changing set of judgements, regarding the significance of the flow of events for a person's well-being. Thus, he shows that secondary cappraisal feeds back to primary appraisal, to mitigate or increase the original threat. He includes **reappraisal** which involves changes in an individual's evaluative judgements. Lazarus regards reappraisal as a feedback process because it involves new information regarding the changing person–environment relationship and its significance for well-being (see Figure 1.1, p3).

Lazarus argues that we must treat the person as an **active agent of change** on the environment as well as a respondent to that environment. We need to give as much attention to describing **transactional relationships** as well as to their causal determinants. These relationships are characterised as much by **change and flux** as by stability and consistency. Hence, it is necessary to observe such relationships as they take place over time.

Thus, to conclude, Lazarus offers a comprehensive and humanistic picture of stress as applied to the individual. He places emphasis upon the continuous transactions between the person and his/her environment which may lead to cognitive appraisals of stress and subsequent patterns of coping. In contrast to the macro approaches of the response and stimulus models in which general factors are considered, the transactional model is a micro approach and operates at the level of the individual. Thus, a transactional approach, in keeping with a humanistic perspective, actively acknowledges that an individual's construals of a situation are of central concern in the understanding of his/her experience of stress. Lazarus distinguishes key factors within the individual and the environment pertaining to stress and coping. Yet, it is important to note that there are also likely to exist a diverse range of factors, particularly regarding the individual, that lie undiscovered, due to the complexity of the human mind. These may operate at different layers of consciousness and within the subconscious and remain abstract. Emphasis upon the individual, the complex nature of cognition and the active, changing interplay between the person and his/her environment regarding stress and coping are highly relevant factors in this study. This is because it is directly concerned with the appraisals of stress and subsequent coping processes amongst individuals with cancer.

The following chapter further develops Lazarus' early work upon coping, by applying it directly to persons with cancer. The work of Weisman (1979) is reviewed and compared with Lazarus' later work upon coping.

2   The concept of coping

Weisman (1979) expands upon Lazarus' earlier writings on coping, by applying the concept directly to persons with cancer. He explored three major facets to coping:

- there is usually a problem from which one seeks relief;
- it involves what one does or does not do regarding the problem, i.e. how one copes;
- the effectiveness, or **not**, of the coping strategy.

Similarly to Lazarus, Weisman accepts that while what one does may be highly individualistic, there are general types of behaviour which cover more specific tactics. Weisman labels these as 'strategies' or 'copes'. He presents a list of copes which can be seen to expand from Lazarus' examples of action tendencies and cognitive manoeuvres. For example, rational inquiry, disengagement, externalisation and suppression. Weisman explains that these strategies often intermingle and they are seldom found by themselves. It can be seen that these 'copes' are real examples from everyday life, thus, they can easily be applied to persons with cancer.

Benner and Wrubel (1989) criticise what they view as Weisman's psychodynamic view of the person as a rational problem-solver, i.e. one who tests reality and assumes total responsibility for his/her feelings and actions. They argue that Weisman views coping in a narrow sense, as a trait/talent, that can be judged in a context-free fashion. Lazarus (1984) similarly criticises the use of coping traits and styles, as individuals are assumed to possess static, stable dispositions. He argues that such classifications underestimate the complexity and variability of actual coping efforts. Lazarus recognises the multidimensional quality of coping processes, i.e. that there is both stability and change. He notes that research to date has focused on stable traits rather than on coping as a process.

Denial

Weisman describes the concept of denial in much more detail than Lazarus' early work, revealing that it is a complex coping strategy. In his opinion, it serves three aims:

- it preserves the *status quo*;

- it simplifies the relationship;
- it eliminates the differences between what was and what will be.

Weisman's analysis of denial goes much further than the original writings of Freud (1924), as he examines five phases of denial: acceptance, elimination, replacement, reorientation and judgement. Weisman emphasises that denial is a process that repudiates what cannot be avoided, often by substituting a more familiar agreeable idea. He states that denial is also a transaction, in that it may be encouraged with the collusion of others (e.g. relatives of a person with terminal illness). Weisman acknowledges that persons with cancer who use denial tend to feel increasingly helpless. Thus, the very process intended to foster wellbeing often undermines vitality and collaboration (e.g. by the isolation of significant others).

Weisman also studies the different orders or degrees of denial: repudiation, disorientation and renunciation. Weisman expands upon the third order of denial which he calls 'middle knowledge'. This occurs when a person with advanced cancer suddenly behaves as if nothing is wrong, despite full knowledge of the illness and its manifestations (i.e. knowing and not knowing at the same time). Such individuals shift back and forth between awareness, coping and denial. He argues that there is no reason to expect a smooth transition from early denial toward pure acceptance. (Compare with the work of Kubler-Ross, see p19.)

'Effective' coping

Weisman attempts to examine what exactly constitutes 'effective' coping. He states that there is no secret formula for good coping that will suit every person with cancer. However, he defines 'good copers' as individuals who avoid avoidance, i.e. do not deny, but confront realities and take appropriate action. They tend to focus on solutions or redefine a problem into a solvable form. 'Good copers' always consider alternatives and maintain open, mutual communication with significant others. They seek and use constructive help, including medical and nursing care, are assertive when necessary and are optimistic.

This sounds very difficult to achieve, especially when a person is first diagnosed as having cancer. In his later comments, Lazarus argues that coping includes efforts to manage stressful demands **regardless** of outcome. Thus, no one strategy is considered inherently better or worse than any other. In this way, denial can be positive when there is nothing constructive the individual can do to overcome harm. Benner and Wrubel similarly propose that often the person confronts more unspecified problems, thus defences, such as denial, allow needed respite and sufficient time to take appropriate action.

Weisman feels that hope is a pre-requisite for 'good' coping and expands further on this concept. He also states that very hopeful individuals set goals for themselves and try to reach them, trusting others when necessary. Weisman views hope as being designed to see people through adversity. He argues that when hopeful people acquire cancer, they are tenacious and resourceful. However, this is clearly a broad generalisation and it is important to realise that there are likely to be many variations, due to the fact that persons with cancer are unique in the ways they adjust to the diagnosis of cancer.

Weisman defines 'poor copers' as individuals who usually feel defeated at the outset. Such individuals insist on helping themselves, thus obtaining minimal support from others. They also tend to deny a great deal, so that it is increasingly difficult to get direct confirmation of distress. Weisman argues that 'poor copers' may adopt a passive attitude of waiting for something to be done rather than adopting an active method of coping. Where 'effective' copers are more inclined to be optimistic, 'poor copers' are generally pessimistic.

There are clear parallels with the description of Weisman's 'poor copers' to the 'unpopular patient' outlined by Stockwell (1980). The unpopular patient is likely to grumble and complain; communicate a dislike of being in hospital; imply that he/she is suffering more than is believed by the nurses and is preoccupied with minor things or demanding attention when others need it. This is in contrast to the patients who nurses enjoy caring for, which parallel Weisman's description of 'good copers'. These patients are able to communicate readily with nurses; able to laugh and joke with nurses; co-operate by helping in the 'get well' process and are determined to do so.

Stockwell argues that this carries implications for nursing care, as the nurses in her study sometimes adopted deterrent behaviour for 'difficult' patients (e.g. ignoring the patient; forgetting his/her requests; refusing gifts and favours; enforcing rules and using sarcasm). In contrast, if the nurses stopped to talk to patients, they were highly likely to choose the patients they most enjoyed caring for.

Benner and Wrubel criticise Weisman for overlooking the relationship between the person and his/her situation, as emphasised by Lazarus' transactional model of stress. They argue that Weisman views hope as a personal trait (i.e. the person is viewed as being morally responsible for all their feelings) and infers personal blame when hope is not available. They conclude that there are major problems with defining some strategies as good and others as bad because an individual's situation is not taken into consideration. Benner and Wrubel label Weisman's approach as an 'outside–in view', which lends itself to 'trivial lists of advice', offering little guidance and understanding of what advice might mean to specific people in specific situations.

Concept of vulnerability

Weisman expands upon the concept of non-coping by linking it with the concept of vulnerability. He defines this as designating different types, degrees and fluctuations of **distress** over time. It is also an implicit measurement of non-coping. Weisman constructed an index of vulnerability to express the **common** types of distress and easily recognised distress signals. He explains that the central core of vulnerability is the condition of helpless uncertainty, which he calls 'existential despair', i.e. concern regarding life and death. There are four main vulnerability variables:

- annihilation (hopelessness)
- alienation (abandonment)
- endangerment (frustration)
- denial

The end point of the scale is directly concerned with extreme reactions of persons with cancer. From these main variables, persons with cancer can be differentiated according to their most prevalent vulnerability factors. Weisman's Index can be regarded as a tool for detecting more extreme possible psychiatric reactions, in keeping with a medical model, as opposed to psychological reactions often experienced by persons with cancer.

Weisman attempted to predict distress amongst persons with cancer. At the time of initial diagnosis and at further intervals, he contrasts psychosocial characteristics of persons (with newly diagnosed cancer) found to be in higher emotional distress (HED) with those of persons found to have lower emotional distress (LED). Overall, HED patients are seen to correspond with 'poor copers', as they are seen to be increasingly pessimistic, have regrets regarding their past and expect little support from family and friends. In contrast, LED patients are seen to correspond with 'good copers', as they are increasingly optimistic and perceive themselves as receiving adequate support.

Weisman's work on the concept of vulnerability is original and highly relevant to persons with cancer. However, it is important to remember that Weisman aims to classify extremes of coping and non-coping. This is similar to a medical model and the focus on classifying people in terms of their illness. It can be seen that in everyday life, there are a wide range of variations between these two poles, as no two persons with cancer are likely to react to a diagnosis of cancer in exactly the same way. As argued by Benner and Wrubel, it is essential to consider the individual's unique world, skills, history, concerns and current circumstances when studying coping patterns. An individual cannot be divorced from his/her situation. This links to the phenomenological perspective, with the emphasis on the meanings an individual ascribes to his/her experiences in everyday life.

Psychosocial staging in cancer

Weisman finally examines critical periods in the life of the person with cancer, which he refers to as the 'psychosocial staging in cancer'. It is original in that it is directly applicable to persons with cancer. (see pp19–20 for parallels with Kubler-Ross.)

Stage I

Weisman calls Stage I the 'essential plight' which consists of two concepts:

- 'Impact distress' concerns what happens at that moment when a person first definitely learns about his/her cancer. He explains that this is an alarming moment, when approximately one third of persons with cancer in his study saw death as a real possibility.
- 'Existential plight proper' goes beyond the impact to the point when primary treatment ends and the person attempts to resume an ordinary life. This second stage, which covers the first one hundred days, includes plight's peak. For some individuals, there

is increased distress and for others, their distress is reduced as the disease progresses. Weisman notes that distress is likely to be proportional to the severity of physiological symptoms.

Stage II

This involves 'mitigation and accommodation' and represents a psychosocial analogue of the established disease. Weisman explains that this stage can last indefinitely. It ranges from those who have early and permanent remission, to those who remain sick or become worse almost as soon as primary (first-time) treatment ends. Thus, it is an extremely wide-ranging stage. It constitutes a stage of adaptation. In this way, signs of 'good coping' are attributes of having mitigated and accommodated to the fact of cancer, with subsequent increased quality of life.

Stage III

This involves 'decline and deterioration'. This sometimes occurs without obvious physiological changes. The person with cancer has reached a point of no return, regardless of their treatment. This leads to a decrease in the person's quality of life.

Stage IV

This involves 'preterminality and terminality'. Preterminality occurs when dying begins. Individuals tend to preterminally yield active responsibility and either ask for help or withdraw from further efforts to help themselves. This represents a time to exchange active strategies for those that depend on passive co-operation.

Weisman's psychosocial staging represents a simplistic view of the differing stages through which the person with cancer passes. For example, it can be seen that not all persons with cancer may experience Stage III, if they are coping effectively with their diagnosis. Likewise, as Weisman admits, some persons with cancer may reach Stage III prematurely, as they may 'give up' completely. Again, it is important to remember that some individuals with cancer may experience these stages at different moments in time, or may not experience any/most of these at all. Thus, Weisman's Stages I to IV are too rigid when judged sequentially. They are much more effective when viewed as possibly occurring at some moment in the lives of individuals with cancer. However, the exact time in which they occur (or do not occur, as the case may be), differs from one individual to another. Lazarus criticises the use of stages which may exert pressure on persons with cancer to comply with these expectations.

Kubler-Ross

Weisman's psychosocial staging of cancer is, however, much more complex than the earlier work of Kubler-Ross (1969). Kubler-Ross' stages are restrictive and relate to some of the stress emotions outlined earlier by Lazarus (e.g. anger, depression). In effect, Kubler-Ross describes primitive forms of coping. Her stages are not as comprehensive as the work of Lazarus on defence mechanisms, but the work was the first of its kind to directly relate to the psychological experience of death and dying.

Denial and isolation

Kubler-Ross states that most persons with terminal illness react to their first awareness of their own possible death by thinking or saying 'no not me, it can't be true'. In contrast to Weisman, she does not include the possible harmful effects of the long-term use of denial.

Anger

Kubler-Ross explains that when the first stage of denial cannot be maintained, it is replaced by feelings of anger, rage, envy and resentment. The anger is displaced in all directions and is also projected onto the environment, as the person finds grievances. This stage can be criticised for its simplicity, as it does not include all possible stress emotions a person with cancer may experience. The person may experience anger at the outset; alternatively they may not experience anger at all. The emotion of anger, in the context of Stage II is not relevant to all persons with terminal illness.

Bargaining

This occurs when the person with cancer believes that they may succeed in entering into some sort of an agreement, which may postpone the inevitable from happening. The person uses manoeuvres to wish for an extension of life. This stage involves a form of defence mechanism first outlined by Freud (1924) and expanded upon by Lazarus. However, it does not include other equally viable defence mechanisms in this stage. Some individuals with cancer may not adopt bargaining as a defence mechanism. Likewise, other individuals may use bargaining at an earlier or later stage.

Depression

This occurs when a person with cancer has increased symptoms and all possible treatment(s) and can no longer 'smile it off'. The person experiences a sense of loss which leads to feelings of depression. Kubler-Ross explains that preparatory depression occurs when a person prepares for the final separation from the world by taking into account impending losses. This stage can be criticised, similar to Stage II, because depression is outlined in isolation from other specific stress emotions, such as anxiety.

Acceptance

Kubler-Ross considers that if a person with cancer has had time to work through the stages, they are neither depressed or angry about their 'fate'. She explains that it is a stage almost void of feelings, as the struggle is over and the person finds peace in the form of acceptance. Kubler-Ross' final stage of acceptance is suspect because, for some persons with cancer, acceptance may be reached much earlier, as explained by Weisman. However, other persons may not reach full acceptance at any time because they wish to continue to fight their disease or to continue to deny their disease. Kubler-Ross' stages present a narrow view of the concept of coping. Some individuals may not 'work through' any of these stages, but may experience some of the concepts outlined in these states at any moment in time, depending upon the person and his/her unique situation.

Thus, to conclude the work upon psychosocial staging, although Weisman presents a much more comprehensive analysis of psychosocial staging than Kubler-Ross, it still tends to limit the wide range of emotions and defences the person with cancer may or may not experience at any given moment in time. To put these emotions and defences into rigid stages, leads to a stereotyped portrayal of the way in which individuals cope with their illness over a period of time.

Coping mechanisms

Lazarus (1984), in his later text, studies appraisal, coping and adaptational outcomes with reference to recent research. He explores how coping mechanisms affect physical and psychological health. He cites increasing evidence that passive acceptance, helplessness and depression tend to be associated with a poorer outlook for survival, than the use of anger and fighting to stay alive or to control one's circumstances. Morris, Greer and Pettingale (1981) found that cancer patients who had attitudes of denial or fighting spirits, as opposed to fatal or helplessness/hopelessness attitudes, were significantly more likely to still be alive. Similarly, DiClemente and Temoshok (1985) found that, amongst persons with malignant melanoma, women with fatalistic attitudes and men with high helplessness/hopelessness scores had an increasingly rapid disease progression over a period of one to two years. They argued that persons who see cancer as a challenge and feel that they have some influence over the disease have better adjustment. Lazarus is careful to note, however, that there are always individual differences in physiological and psychological responses, as opposed to a uniform generalised human response as outlined by Selye (1957) (see p1).

Coping rate system

Morris, Buckley and Blake (1986) developed a useful rating system relating to coping and cancer by adapting Lazarus' work on coping. They were directly concerned with the cognitive responses of individuals with cancer. From their study, they identified three main types of responses which were called 'A' appraisal statements, 'B' and 'C' strategies.

'A' appraisal statements

These consist of persons' evaluations of their cancer diagnosis. These evaluations of cancer were made in terms of severity, anticipated impact on their lives and their emotional response to it. Some individuals also made attributions of their cancer to a variety of causes. Morris, Buckley and Blake distinguished ten evaluations. For example, 'lacks concern about the diagnosis', 'passively accepts the diagnosis'. The statements are directly relevant to Lazarus' concept of cognitive appraisal of a situation (see p4). However, it must be remembered that each individual appraises a situation (in this case, the diagnosis of cancer) differently. Thus, although Morris, Buckley and Blake devised ten appraisal statements, there may well be many more and some may not even fit into these appraisals. They attempted to discover the **main** appraisal statements expressed by their sample of newly diagnosed persons with cancer.

'B' strategies

Morris, Buckley and Blake were then able to distinguish nine ways in which persons with cancer appear to manipulate their thinking about a diagnosis of cancer, in order to reduce its mental impact. For example, by blocking, disassociating, partialising, assigning control and using humour. These are, in effect, examples of defence mechanisms first outlined by Freud and later expanded upon by Lazarus. The above examples differ from those given by Lazarus and Weisman. Thus, it is clearly possible that the person with cancer may use (albeit unconsciously) a broad range of defence mechanisms in order to cope with their diagnosis of cancer.

'C' strategies

These consist of six statements which describe ways in which individuals encouraged themselves to think positively about their lives, without necessarily mentally reducing the potential harm associated with a cancer diagnosis. All contain implications for future action, e.g. using religion and encouraging a positive mental set. These strategies are a different form of direct-action tendencies first outlined by Lazarus. They do not consist of ways in which the individual physically acts against the threat. Instead, they consist of ways in which the individual psychologically acts directly by thinking through positive psychological means of coping with the threat. Individuals undertaking 'C' strategies would be viewed as 'good copers' by Weisman as they adopt a positive outlook regarding their cancer diagnosis. From these appraisals, Morris, Buckley and Blake have attempted to generate hypotheses regarding the main psychological responses to a diagnosis of cancer, using their rating method and categories developed from their previous work, e.g. a fighting spirit, denial, stoic acceptance, helplessness and hopelessness. Their main aim is to provide others with a means of defining the above responses in their own work. The 'C' strategies hypothesis is the least useful in that it presents a tightly-knit group of responses, as opposed to 'A' appraisal statements which allow much more freedom of choice and illustrate a range of different individual responses to a diagnosis of cancer.

Conclusion

To conclude, Weisman has developed Lazarus' earlier core of knowledge regarding the concept of coping by applying it directly to persons with cancer. His work upon the concepts of denial, vulnerability and psychosocial staging allow deeper insights into coping patterns amongst persons with cancer. However, his work verges at times towards a trait approach, indicative of a medical model, due to his concern with types and dispositions regarding coping and persons with cancer. This leads to the development of stereotypes of coping patterns amongst persons with cancer.

This may be of use in clinical practice, for health care professionals to detect those individuals with cancer experiencing problems with their coping patterns. However, it is essential that nurses, in particular within their support role, appreciate the rich complexity and diversity of coping amongst persons with cancer and adopt a respectful, empathic, non-critical stance towards individuals' coping methods, i.e. a humanistic approach. This reflects Lazarus' transactional model, in which he focuses upon coping processes as they actually occur in life stress. Lazarus criticises the dearth of descriptive studies which explore how a person actually handles a particular harm/threat or challenge over time. This relates to the phenomenological perspective and the importance of describing the meanings individuals give to their life experiences.

3 Health research regarding the concept of stress and persons with cancer

The following areas of health care research have been examined in such a way as to link directly to Lazarus' transactional approach to stress and to the research topic:

- A broad overview of the nature of cancer itself, including people's attitudes towards cancer.
- An analysis of health care literature on the main concerns facing the person with cancer and his/her significant others.

Attitudes towards cancer

It is important initially to focus on the nature of cancer itself, in order to establish why it is perceived as being a stress phenomenon for many individuals. Generally, cancer is seen as an epidemic; the disease people fear most. Deeley (1979) argues that cancer, suffering and death are either synonymous or associated, spread to others and become an accepted fact. He explains that especially where knowledge is deficient (for many people there is a general lack of basic information), there is a readier acceptance of fatal and/or adverse circumstances. This is likely to be due to the associated fear of the unknown for many individuals. For example, the media help to portray a person with cancer as suffering enormous pain and being merely an image of his/her former self, yet stoically fighting on. It can be seen that such images are extremely powerful.

Attitudes are made up of a mixture of basic ideas, hearsay, personal experience and historical events. It can be seen throughout history that there has existed many scourges of mankind (e.g. tuberculosis, yellow fever and leprosy) that produce the same attitude of mind we now find with cancer. The control of these scourges has changed attitudes slowly (Deeley, 1979). Thus, there is the need for a drastic change to take place in treatment (i.e. one which leads to recovery of most persons) before marked changes in attitudes occur. Even then, Deeley concedes that attitudes lag behind medical advances and it sometimes takes a generation before ideas change.

In the case of cancer, not all persons are cured. Doyal (1983) claims that, overall, survival rates have not improved to any great extent over the last thirty years (although specific cancers have shown reduced mortality due to new treatments, e.g. childhood leukaemia and Hodgkin's disease). It is not surprising, therefore, that attitudes of fear are widespread. Many individuals only tend to be aware of cancer when a person dies. They tend to forget that cancer is a name for a whole group of diseases.

Cancer is a subject about which few people, including doctors, can think about without emotion. It is often difficult for those doctors whose ethos is that of a curative role, as they see cancer as a failure on their part. In many cases this leads to feelings of fear and depression (Mitchell, 1979).

Allegory, myth and legend

Pugsley and Pardoe (1988) note the 'unique air of fear' for a person when a diagnosis of cancer is made. Their sociological analysis of the impact of cancer helps to explore the complex human reasoning behind the emotion of fear. They explain that one method of attempting to cope with any phenomenon that is perceived as powerful and life-threatening is to attempt to understand it using allegory, myth and legend. Their analysis of the myths of cancer capture the intensity and breadth of the emotion fear which is often experienced by individuals.

The alien within

The first myth outlined is that of 'the alien within', i.e. it is believed by many persons that cancer is not a disease at all, but an alien entity that lives independently inside an individual's body. In this way, it is thought to lie dormant until the person experiences shock. Thus, once awakened, it starts to grow inside the body until it kills the person. This myth reflects the commonly held view that a stressful occurrence often acts as a precursor to a serious illness such as cancer.

Wages of sin

The second myth, 'wages of sin', reflects the frequently held assumption that the illness is punishment for past sins. Concepts of guilt and its expiation through suffering are commonplace. It is likely that the view of 'wages of sin' is much more likely to hold sway for those individuals with religious beliefs.

Contagion

The third view, 'contagion', is the commonly held belief that cancer is in some way catching. People with cancer are often shunned and are objects of practices of decontamination (Sontag, 1979).

Family myths

Knowledge of family history, including myths, is strong when a family is faced with a crisis such as cancer. Whether cancer is 'in the family' is important, as persons will often say they expected to have cancer as it is 'in the family'. This reflects Johnson's (1988) hereditary theory as a common theory of causality; that individuals tend to base theories of cancer on personal experience.

Pugsley and Pardoe's sociological analysis reveals the importance of exploring an individual's views on the nature of cancer, as they play a crucial role in how the individual reacts to, and subsequently copes with, a diagnosis of cancer.

Thus, many people tend to have a pessimistic outlook towards cancer, indeed often a sense of associated hopelessness. In general, individuals tend to overestimate the number of cancer deaths, underestimate the number of 'cured' (i.e. those in remission) and believe early detection and treatment have little effect on prognosis. Thus, the attitudes of the majority of individuals are 'over-pessimistic'.

Individuals also tend to give anecdotal details of individuals who have had cancer — **'It was cancer you know'** — in hushed tones. Cancer becomes a taboo, a morbid subject, not to be spoken about at social gatherings. Some individuals have 'cancer phobia', they worry about developing cancer, e.g. a woman with a lump in her breast asks **'Is it cancer?'** straightaway. Some people feel pity for the person with cancer and their family, yet also feel relieved that they have not got it (Deeley, 1979).

Cultural meanings of cancer

The association of cancer, death and suffering held by many individuals is carefully analysed by Parker (1981), who explores the cultural meanings of cancer. He argues that death and suffering are taboo in our society for a variety of reasons:

- A gradual loss over time of traditional religious beliefs, which gave a central place to death and suffering. In contrast, a trend is increasingly moving towards secularised scientific orientations by many individuals, with promised cure and freedom from suffering. In this context, it can be easily be seen how death and suffering have become counter evidence to the illusion of progress.

- The associated medicalisation and specialisation in care of the sick tends to separate them from common daily experience. Thus, few persons are likely to have first hand experience of illness and suffering.

- An increasingly consumer-oriented, materialistic focus of societal values with the replacement of old with 'brand new', de-emphasises death and avoids loss. As a result, individuals are likely to appraise death and suffering as stressful experiences and, subsequently, require much support to cope when faced with such situation.

- The current association of good health and cleanliness as a cultural obsession with youth, i.e. images of 'clean and shining bodies'. This, again, leads to avoidance when faced with the contrast of death as the disintegration and decaying of the body.

Parker thus presents a vivid analysis of generalised western cultural themes in relation to cancer as a symbol of death and suffering:

> *'The societal battle against cancer is then seen as the struggle to resist acceptance of the inevitability in life of death, decay and decomposition.'*

Although these overall trends cannot account for individual differences, they nevertheless play a significant role in the development of attitudes amongst individuals with regard to the notions of death, suffering and cancer.

Negative views amongst nurses

Several studies over the last eleven years have shown that attitudes of fear and gloom are not limited to the general public. The majority of nurses are also generally pessimistic regarding the number of deaths caused by cancer. Some trained and more experienced nurses hold a more optimistic view of cancer, but they are in the minority (Elkind, 1982). Most nurses consider it at least sometimes true that treatment can do more harm than good (Elkind, 1981). Such a negative view can easily be transferred from nurse to patient, with ill effects upon the latter (Whelan, 1984). We need to ask ourselves whether nurses who express negative views about cancer are realistically able to motivate the public to undertake preventive care regarding cancer.

Elkind (1982) asked nurses to select the most alarming of a series of serious conditions (e.g. rheumatoid arthritis, coronary heart disease, chronic bronchitis, schizophrenia, cancer of the stomach). The largest proportion of nurses selected cancer of the stomach. Elkind also noted that the less professional experience the nurse had with cancer nursing, the more likely she was to choose cancer of the stomach as the most alarming. Elkind concludes that nurses tend to share the fear of cancer felt by women in general, but it may be modified by education or experience.

Attitude awareness

Craytor and Fass (1982) developed a teaching module to help nurses and other health care professionals view cancer and cancer care in a more positive manner, and also to view themselves as better able to undertake cancer care. The module consists of developing awareness of attitudes, self and cancer nursing with eighteen objectives as behavioural outcomes to be achieved by the learner, using a self-paced approach and small group interaction. They found that post module nurses in their study revealed more positive attitudes regarding cancer.

Education is an essential factor in order to bring about changes in attitudes towards cancer. Health educationalists need to have a better understanding of the nature of individuals' beliefs about cancer and the relationship with their health and illness behaviour. At present, given the above information upon attitudes towards cancer, it is highly likely that an individual recently diagnosed as having cancer will perceive it as a stressful phenomenon. As a result, it is important for the cancer nurse to carry out a thorough psychosocial assessment of a person's perceptions of stress in order to help promote effective psychosocial adjustment to the diagnosis of cancer.

Psychological concerns

Much of the health care literature upon cancer nursing over the last 15 years has acknowledged the prevalence of negative attitudes and has also attempted to explore the major concerns facing the person with cancer. The following section includes a concise analysis of the more recent and most relevant research.

The work of Maguire acts as a framework for this section. He has made a significant contribution to the development of knowledge regarding psychosocial care of the person with cancer. His perspective, as a psychiatrist, is clearly a medical one; nevertheless, several articles aimed for a nursing audience (1985a, 1985c) usefully outline the main concerns of the person with cancer. Thus, he attempts to assess the psychological impact of cancer.

Uncertainty

Uncertainty is a main concern because cancer can recur at any time. The disease does not always follow a straightforward course. Thus, doctors may establish certain progressive patterns, but the exact course of the disease differs greatly from one individual to another and is dependent on multiple variables, i.e. physiological, psychological and social factors (Maguire, 1985a).

Illness is always with them or, if dormant, is potentially lurking just around the corner. Thus, the fear of recurrence is of major concern to the person with cancer. There are many uncertainties facing a person with cancer regarding life itself, significant others and work. Uncertainty regarding diagnosis and outcome is a central theme of psychosocial adjustment in persons newly diagnosed with cancer (Bond, 1982). Uncertainty is a cognitive state that occurs in a situation where the decision maker is unable to assign definitive values to objects and events, and/or is unable to accurately predict outcomes (Mishel *et al*, 1984).

Loss of an expected future

In conjunction with feelings of uncertainty, there also exists a sense of loss of an expected future (Holmes, 1985). As a result, the person with cancer is not able to plan far ahead and has the possible threat of a disabling chronic illness, mutilation, loss of an important body part, loss of self-worth, pain and even death itself. All these threats, excluding death, may well involve significant physiological and psychosocial changes in the individual's previous lifestyle (Welch McCaffrey, 1985).

There is a tendency for our society today to be future-oriented. People without cancer look forward to the time when, for example, their children are older and the house is paid for. In contrast, the orientation of the person with cancer is often directed towards survival rather than future joy. This may accentuate the feeling of being different (Northouse, 1981).

Preoccupation with death

The person with cancer is likely to be frequently concerned with the prospect of death. A study of cancer nurses with cancer revealed that most respondents spent much personal time thinking about death after their diagnosis (Welch McCaffrey, 1984). This is not surprising given many people's attitudes to cancer. Another study of depression in elderly persons with cancer found that one of the five most common areas of concern associated with depressive symptoms was death. Therefore, it is necessary to know how a person has coped with loss/death in the past and whether he/she experienced significant depression at these times (Goldberg and Cullen, 1986).

For some individuals, a main area of concern is the fear of the process of dying, (i.e. the fear of an extremely painful death, the loss of control over physical functions and the fear of being alone) (Fallowfield, 1988). However, this is more likely to apply to persons in the advanced stages of cancer who are facing the prospect of death.

Search for meaning

The person with cancer is also concerned with a search for meaning. He/she may ask him/herself, 'Why me?' 'Why now?' The person may then feel a sense of failure. He/she may also view the onset of cancer as a fault of his/her personality, or as a flawed lifestyle. Some individuals may even feel that their bodies have let them down, by developing a serious chronic illness (Maguire, 1985a).

Sense of isolation

Maguire writes of an associated sense of isolation, i.e. a feeling of social loss. Northouse (1981) quotes a patient who explained:

> *'I sometimes feel that the whole world is over there and I'm at the opposite side of the field watching everyone else.'*

The uncertainty regarding the outcome and seriousness of the disease is difficult for family. Thus, the lack of open communication may be awkward, leading to embarrassment and a significant decrease in the frequency and length of contacts. The person with cancer may also feel that they are completely alone in coping with their worries.

Buckalew's personal account (1982) of her admission to a cancer hospital vividly recalls how she experienced a great sense of isolation at night and found that this was greatly relieved by telephoning her husband.

Many families are unable to discuss death, hence communication may break down and, subsequently, the person mourns the loss of significant relationships (Goldberg and Cullen, 1986). A study found that out of one hundred healthy people, approximately three quarters would avoid contact with a friend who had cancer. Amongst persons with breast cancer, over half of the sample felt people avoided them and three quarters of the sample expressed a lack of understanding from family and friends. This served to heighten their feelings of social isolation (Peters-Golden, 1982).

Effect on the family

The reaction of a person's significant others is crucial to that person's effective adjustment to his/her illness and the ability to maintain close interpersonal relationships with family and friends is most important. A diagnosis of cancer may be very difficult for relatives to accept and this may lead to conflicts and direct avoidance of open communication with the person. Yet family may well have feelings of deep concern towards the person (Mishel, *et al*, 1984).

In some relationships, the development of cancer in one of the partners strengthens their bonds together, whilst in others it has negative effects. It may also involve a change in roles, e.g. the significant others may have to become increasingly active in a variety of domestic chores. Thus, it does often mean increased work for family members, who may become physically and mentally exhausted over a period of time (Stromberg and Wright, 1984).

There are possible changes in behaviour of family members. For example, a young adolescent may take the place of his/her father who is sick, or he/she may retreat back to childhood and refuse to take on this new role. Thus, a central concern for the person with cancer is the impact of the diagnosis on family and friends.

Feelings of helplessness

The individual with cancer may often worry about how his/her family is coping, yet feel helpless to do anything active to alleviate the situation. The social dependency affecting the person with cancer has been found to be inversely associated with quality of life (Young and Longman, 1983). Feelings of helplessness are often experienced by the person with cancer and are related to the illness itself. This is largely due to the fact that there is little the individual can actively do to prevent a recurrence or spread of the illness.

Attention is also drawn to the person's concern regarding finances. For example, if the person is the major breadwinner and is no longer able to work, he/she is placing a financial burden onto his/her spouse and children, due to loss of income. The person may feel a sense of failure regarding inability to work and meet obligations. Subsequently, family relationships are likely to be affected (Stromberg and Wright, 1984; Welch McCaffrey, 1984).

Many individuals have a feeling of dependency which is a direct cause of concern. Persons with cancer often have a lack of choice in the decisions regarding their treatment and day-to-day living. This may lead to feelings of loss of control over physiological function; a sense of the body being out of control. This is seen in varying degrees in hospital as health professionals (albeit sometimes unwittingly) 'take over' and the person with cancer becomes dependent on them for his/her treatment and care (Mishel *et al*, 1984).

Effects of treatment

A major concern of the cancer patient is the effects of treatment. The surgical removal of a limb has been shown to have radical effects on the individual (Maguire *et al*, 1980a). Chemotherapy often causes nausea and vomiting. Thus, stimuli associated with chemotherapy can also elicit nausea and vomiting. Anticipatory nausea and vomiting occurs in approximately a quarter of all persons undergoing courses of chemotherapy (Mohrer *et al*, 1984). A study of conditioned averse responses in persons receiving chemotherapy found that increased levels of anxiety led to an increased incidence in anticipatory nausea and vomiting. Highly anxious persons are likely to be extremely vigilant to stimuli associated with the chemotherapy setting (Burish and Carey, 1986). This can lead to the development of conditioned responses. Buckalew (1982) recalls her personal experiences of chemotherapy and explains that her knowledge of the inevitable side effects made her 'gag' instinctively as she walked onto the ward.

There is considerable evidence to suggest that the greater the toxicity of the drugs given, the more likely the person is to experience increased emotional distress and a poorer quality of life. Nausea and vomiting may be so intolerable that persons refuse treatment. Literature on American treatment centres notes that 80% of centres had 10% of persons who refused further treatment due to the distress of nausea and vomiting (Fallowfield, 1988).

Radiotherapy often causes individuals to feel lethargic for several weeks after treatment has finished and this often causes depression in many people (Devlen, 1984). A study of persons receiving radiotherapy postmastectomy found that they experienced stress due to the practicalities associated with treatment, i.e. the daily trips to the hospital (sometimes long distances) and the disruption of daily family and work routines. The daily visits serve as a daily reminder to the person that he/she has cancer. In addition, the relatively impersonal nature of radiotherapy, the few contacts with professional staff and being left alone in a room with a huge machine can be disturbing (Silberfarb, 1978). The effects of long periods of waiting and talking to other seriously ill persons often has a profoundly depressing effect, e.g. a person having curative treatment who fears that he/she shares the fate of those having palliative treatment; the fears people harbour regarding radiotherapy (some individuals worry that the radiotherapy used to treat cancer paradoxically causes cancer) (Fallowfield, 1988). Thus, it can be seen that there are a diverse range of concerns facing persons undergoing cancer treatment.

Psychiatric morbidity

The side-effects of treatment can represent **potential** obstacles to effective psychological adaptation. They can contribute to substantial psychiatric morbidity associated with the cancer diagnosis and treatment.

Maguire gives a definition of depressive illness which focuses on the physiological effects of depression. Thus, a person who reports that he/she has been feeling persistently low (approximately for over four weeks), feels miserable and is 'fed up', to the extent which represents a significant and obvious departure from normal mood, is said to be depressed. The person also often lacks energy and appetite and experiences loss in weight and interest. This is clearly a medical definition which fails to consider the diverse range of possible psychosocial factors involved.

'Anxiety state' is described in a similar fashion. The person worries endlessly regarding their predicament. The person cannot stop thinking about his/her concerns, nor can he/she be distracted by other people. The individual is persistently unable to relax. The key somatic signs include sweating, difficulty in sleeping, irritability and reduced concentration. Again, it can be seen that Maguire is primarily concerned with physiological effects, indicative of a medical model. Weisman (1979) counter argues that 'every person with cancer is not simply anxious or depressed, as people are too complex to sloganise about them.' Each individual with cancer is a unique being and, as such, the nature and intensity of individuals' problems vary.

However, it is useful to study the prevalence of depressive and anxiety states amongst individuals with cancer. With regard to specific cancers, Maguire *et al's* study of women with mastectomies revealed that one in four developed severe psychological problems within the first postoperative year. Similar results have been found with persons with colostomies (McDonald *et al*, 1985). Studies have also found that a substantial minority of persons develop severe psychological problems during and after the use of combination chemotherapy, due to the number and severity of side effects. Radiotherapy also causes some people to develop depression for several months after treatment (Devlen, 1984).

In studies of persons with lymphoma, it has been found that psychological morbidity bore no relation to the type or stage of disease, but rather to the toxicity of the treatment. Devlen (1984) expresses concern regarding the proportion of persons, postchemotherapy, who continued to experience irritability, tiredness and an appreciable loss of libido, and the proportion of persons free of disease and no longer receiving treatment, who failed to return to work or resume normal activities. She found that those who had returned to work were assigned to a lower level of responsibility and some individuals developed illness behaviour. Thus, she concludes that a substantial number of people pay a high price for the prospect of long-term survival and ways of reducing this cost need to be found.

There is often an increase in psychological morbidity in persons with advanced disease, due to an increase in unpleasant symptoms. However, approximately two in every three persons suffering psychological morbidity have only moderate disease symptoms and one third of these persons experience severe psychological symptoms which require intervention by a psychiatrist (Maguire, 1988c). Although psychological morbidity occurs in a minority of persons (and Maguire offers a detailed medically-biased approach to this subject), it is nevertheless useful to consider the possible extreme reactions a person with cancer may experience.

Body image and sexual problems

Persons with cancer can suffer from three types of body image problems, either singly or in combination. A woman who has lost a breast may report a heightened self-consciousness which may be so acute that she begins to avoid people and stays off work. For another woman, the key problem may be that she cannot accept that she is less than whole. She experiences lack of confidence and self-esteem.

The loss of a breast may also have a profound effect on a woman's feelings of being feminine and attractive to others. Up to 20% of women undergoing mastectomy develop one or more of these body image problems which can be disruptive to their social functioning and personal relationships. A greater proportion of persons with colostomies (over 30%) experience body image problems. These often stem from the individual's concern that his/her bag will be visible to other people, could leak, smell, burst, make a noise, be offensive to others, as well as interfere with his/her sexual relationship (McDonald *et al*, 1985).

Between a quarter and a third of persons with a mastectomy develop sexual problems. When treatment involves surgery which damages the genital organs or the necessary nerve supply, sexual problems are much more common. Radiotherapy affects the ovaries which may cause oestrogen deficiency and lead to a lack of lubrication. The use of chemotherapy can also cause infertility (Maguire, 1985a).

Welch McCaffrey (1984) creates a more holistic approach by studying the concept of sexuality as opposed to specific sexual problems. In her study of cancer nurses with cancer, she found that sexuality was an important issue for many respondents. For example, nurses who were single were afraid of the prospect of sterility, of explaining surgical scars and finding accepting partners. Married nurses were worried regarding the possibility of being unable to start a family and the impact of their disfigurement on their marriage. Welch Mccaffrey makes a distinction between sexuality problems involving external alterations (e.g. physical disfigurement and body image problems) and internal changes (e.g. removal of reproductive organs, functional difficulties during intercourse, dealing with sterility and mourning over the inability to have children). This study provides a more in-depth account of the diverse effects that cancer and its treatment has upon the sexuality of the person.

To summarise, it can be seen that there are a wide range of concerns that face the person with cancer and his/her significant others. Maguire's articles give a clear outline of the main concerns facing the person with cancer. However, for a more in-depth humanistic approach which explores the wide-ranging effects upon the individual and his/her significant others, it is essential to explore relevant psychological theory. This is much more likely to give a valid insight into the life of the person with cancer in relation to individual perceptions of stress (see Chapters 5, 6 and 7).

4   The psychological support role of the cancer nurse

rea regarding psychological aspects of nursing care
sses the support role of the cancer nurse. Difficulty with
formation is one of the main expressed concerns of the
family members of adult persons with cancer. Respondents often find
it difficult to obtain concrete answers from doctors and to elicit the
patient's daily progress from nurses (Wright and Dyck, 1984;
Wiltshaw, 1986).

This study concentrates on the support role of the cancer nurse.
There has been much nursing literature over the last 15 years on the
importance of effective communication between the person with
cancer and his/her family and the nursing staff.

Patterns of nurse-client communication

It is important to study the patterns of communication between
nurses and persons with cancer, in order to determine whether the
nursing staff detect the problems of persons with cancer and whether
persons with cancer feel able to express their worries or problems
(Maguire, 1978).

Maguire (1985c) argues that up to 80% of persons with cancer
suffering from psychological morbidity go unrecognised or
untreated. He found that depression amongst individuals on a
cancer ward was regarded by the nursing staff as a natural response
to cancer and its treatment. He refers to this as the use of
normalisation techniques, i.e. it was not regarded as warranting
intervention unless a person became particularly unco-operative and
withdrawn.

Several key studies of communication between nurses and
persons with cancer are critical of the supportive role of the nurse,
which should ideally include the ability to detect and monitor the
problems of persons with cancer. Bond (1982) is of the opinion that
nurses give a low level of attention to the social and psychological
aspects of illness. She found that nurses rarely interacted for longer
than about three minutes with persons not requiring physical care.
Maguire considers that one of the main reasons for failure to detect
hidden psychological morbidity amongst women who were

postmastectomy was that nurses did not routinely inquire about the persons' psychological adjustment. He refers to this as distancing tactics, as nurses assume that persons will disclose problems. Thus, nurses rarely inquire directly regarding persons' adjustment. This is seen as part of a professional bias towards the physical symptoms of illness and leads the person with cancer to believe that the nurse's prime concern is with the person's physical wellbeing. When the nursing staff ask a person how he/she feels, the person interprets this as an inquiry regarding physical health. If a person risks disclosure about an emotional problem, some nurses may engage in a variety of diverting tactics, e.g. attempting to brush away the problem with premature or false reassurances (i.e. jolly the person along), ignore the person's words and change the topic of conversation or avoid entering into conversation with the individual (Bond, 1982; Maguire, 1985b). If a person with cancer had an emotional outburst which influenced other persons, the nurses would move the offending person or ask the individual concerned to control such outbursts.

Many nurses fail to clarify responses and give inadequate information which often misleads the person with cancer. It is important to establish how a person has been affected by the information given to him/her regarding the diagnosis and treatment, and the individual's perceptions. Similarly, it is helpful to ask the person what is understood from the explanations given, as anxiety often leads to poor concentration and difficulty in encoding information.

Clearly, these techniques used by nurses can be described as effectively blocking communication. They are factors which 'get in the way' of free and full communication. Dimbleley and Burton (1988) use the analogy of a filter to gain the impression of obstruction in the mind, as the individual attempts to make sense of the information. They explain that psychological barriers consist of attitudes, beliefs and values which shape what we say before we say it and affect how we interpret what others say to us. These barriers to communication described by Dimbleley and Burton are represented in Fig. 4.1.

Context
Mechanical barriers

Assumptions   Assumptions

Experience   Sender – encode – message – decode – receiver Experience

Beliefs   Beliefs

Semantic barriers

Psychological barriers

Figure 4.1 Barriers to communication (Dimbleby & Burton 1988)

This model can be applied to the blocking tactics of cancer nurses, which may operate at any or all of the three modes of barriers, i.e. mechanical, semantic and psychological.

Some nurses attempt to maintain an emotional distance. They also take the view that they are acting in the best interests of the person, as the less the problem is discussed, the less upset the person will become. Maguire explains that nurses believe it unwise to go looking for problems by directly asking about a person's psychological welfare. This may lead to a person asking difficult questions, which may prove impossible for the nurse to handle. Many nurses also fear that the person may reveal strong emotions which may cause distress in the nurse concerned. Thus, stress is a two way interaction. One person is likely to influence and be influenced by the other.

In order to avoid such a situation, both patients and nursing staff pretend that persons with cancer are coping well emotionally. Nurses tend to ignore crucial verbal and non-verbal cues, which persons give about their problems. For example, individuals who give no overt signs of distress which staff can recognise, deny their illness and do not ask many questions, are seen as coping well because their behaviour does not pose any threats. In contrast, those persons with emotional outbursts disturb the *status quo* of the ward and create difficulties for the nursing staff.

Most nurses are worried about their own emotional survival. Nurses are under pressure and fear that if they routinely inquire regarding a person with cancer's psychological wellbeing, it may not only significantly increase their workload, but they may not be able to cope. They fear becoming emotionally drained and, hence, they have a tendency to selectively avoid persons. Menzies (1960) describes the structure of nursing as an organisation (e.g. task allocation acts as a defence mechanism allowing nurses to remain detached from persons).

When turning to the question 'Do nurses act as support agents for persons with cancer?', it is not surprising to find that few persons tend to talk to the nursing staff about their psychological wellbeing (Baum and Jones, 1979). Studies reveal that half of the persons with cancer in an outpatient radiotherapy department who were anxious or depressed did **not** express their feelings. Of the persons postmastectomy affected by depression, few disclosed their problems to anyone concerned with their care. As a result, few women received the help they needed to resolve their problems.

Approximately 90% of the patients in Bond's study reported that they would have wanted a discussion regarding their overall situation. Yet, they did not feel that the nursing staff were appropriate. In Holmes' study (1985), many persons with cancer linked feelings of isolation with an inability to talk to the nurses. Bond explains that there appeared to be a reluctance on the individuals' part to disclose personal feelings. She gives the following probable reasons for this:

- Patients see the nursing staff as being too busy to concern themselves with anything other than physical needs. The individuals with cancer feel they are not entitled to take up any more of the nurses' time with 'other' worries.

- Patients see the nurses as appearing cheerful and energetic and fear that the nurses may be unsympathetic to their problems.

- An admission of problems may appear silly and unco-operative to others. Persons see others apparently coping well and attempt to maintain a similar appearance so as not to feel isolated and unco-operative.

- Patients attempt to protect the staff as well as relatives by maintaining silence about their emotional worries.

Bond, therefore, concludes that it is likely that persons with cancer rely on others rather than nurses as an outlet for their emotional difficulties.

An American study found that approximately 80% of a sample of persons with cancer were supported by personal friends and family. Of these persons, only 38% received professional support in conjunction with family/friend support. Only 25% of the sample said that nurses were a significant source of support. Two per cent of the sample identified a professional (i.e. a nurse or a doctor) as the sole source of support (Bullough, 1981). Clearly, nurses have not yet established themselves in the public mind as a group that can, and do, give emotional support to persons with cancer.

Fellow patients play an important supportive role. Johnston (1982) found that other patients are more accurate in estimating the number of worries a person has and tend to be more sensitive in detecting what those worries are. This is in contrast to nurses with responsibility for the person. These nurses tend to over-estimate the number of worries of the individual with cancer and are likely to mistakenly address worries which the person is not experiencing.

Several key British studies suggest that most nurses are not yet equipped to give emotional support to the person with cancer because the nurses find it extremely difficult and stressful to do so. It has been acknowledged that the stress amongst nurses working with persons with advanced cancer is only slightly less than the stress experienced by new widows, and actually higher than women commencing radiation treatment for breast cancer (Vachon, 1978). Therefore, it is clear that the stress levels of nurses is a significant factor which affects their patterns of communication.

It appears that some cancer nurses are failing to give emotional support to persons with cancer. Instead, these nurses tend to focus solely on the physical needs related to the persons' illness and treatment. This lack of support is usually associated with a much poorer psychological outcome for the individual with cancer.

The literature points to inadequacy in the current nurse's education, training and communication skills. Rather than being a subject that is taught, communication is simply regarded as an accumulation of experience. As a result, common sense methods are used with tactics and routines learnt through experiences and observation. Bond criticises this unbalanced approach, as it completely cuts off possible alternative practices and learning strategies.

It has been argued that communication is a skill which, in the same way as any other type of skill, needs to be learnt carefully before it can be applied in practice. Communication skills need to be introduced in basic education and developed further in postbasic courses. Tutors need to compare the proportion of teaching time devoted to meeting the physical needs of persons with cancer, with the amount of time given to meeting persons' psychosocial needs (Bridge and Clark, 1981).

Nurses working on cancer wards need to have training in the psychological aspects of cancer. They would then be able to develop specialist communication skills for interviewing and assessing. This would include examining the psychosocial areas of a person's history. Nurses would be able to monitor an individual's emotional adjustment to his/her illness on a daily basis, by making explicit enquiries as to how the individual is coping at specific moments in time (Maguire *et al* 1980).

Maguire gives the following examples of routine screening questions, in order to detect and monitor problems following mutilating surgery:

- How have you been feeling since your operation?
- Do you often feel especially miserable or worried?
- How have you been sleeping?
- Have you found it easy to adapt to everyday life?
- Are you as active socially as you were before surgery?
- What about your relationship with your partner — has that been affected? (Have you resumed love-making yet?)
- How do you feel about your breast loss?
- How do you feel when you catch sight of your chest?
- Have you had any phantom sensations or pain?
- How do you feel about your prosthesis?
- Are there any other problems?

It can be seen that the above questions are open-ended, thereby encouraging the person to voice his/her fears. Specialist communication skills would enable nurses to detect any evidence of symptoms of psychiatric morbidity on admission to hospital and, subsequently, to act upon their findings.

Maguire *et al* (1980) found that a specialist (mastectomy) nurse, who assessed persons with cancer in an outpatient department, detected latent psychiatric symptoms in 90% of those persons who subsequently developed psychiatric problems. The rest of the nursing staff, who had not received any specialist training, failed to detect any psychiatric symptoms in these persons. The cancer specialist acts as a catalyst and as a role model for the rest of the nursing staff. In Britain, unfortunately, such posts are still rare in cancer wards.

Presurgical counselling is now beginning to be increasingly recognised as an essential feature of longer-term planned intervention. Studies support the value of counselling. Half an hour of non-directive counselling preoperatively can have a lasting effect on psychological adjustments. Sometimes, **ten** minutes may be sufficient for someone to talk about his/her most important worries and this investment of time could well prevent a possible crisis at a later date (Burton and Parker, 1988; Moorey, 1988).

Counselling is one of the more complex communication skills. MacLeod Clark places various components of communication into a hierarchy (see Fig 4.2) and concludes that, at present, nurses are more able to use those skills at the top of the hierarchy, but are unable to employ the more in-depth skills at the bottom, which have to be learned and practised.

Often, the need for information, advice and explanation is more acute during the early stages of illness. Information-giving has been shown to be beneficial in reducing physiological and psychological discomfort and increasing feelings of personal control. However, individual preferences for the amount of information should be respected (McCleod Clark and Sims, 1988).

```
information

        advice

             reassurance

                    discussion of diagnosis,
                    treatment and prognosis

                           discussion of feelings

                                  counselling
```

Fig. 4.2 Hierarchy of communication skills (MacLeod Clark, 1981)

There are various strategies that have been put forward to help nurses in the assessment of psychosocial wellbeing of persons' with cancer. Morrow *et al*'s (1978) Psychosocial Adjustment to Illness Scale consists of seven areas of adjustment: health care orientation, vocational environment, domestic environment, sexual relationships, family relationships, social environment and psychological distress. It represents a systematic assessment of a person's adjustment to illness. However, it is complex and nurses require training in order to use it effectively. Izsak and Medalie's scale (1971) is much simpler to use. They map out the physical, psychological and social progress of persons with particular types of cancer and cover recognised key topics.

Welch McCaffrey (1984) argues that nursing assessment of persons with cancer is essential. Before the problem can be treated, the cancer nurse needs to identify it accurately. This requires the nurse to take an active role in interpreting the presence of stress in each individual. However, due to the complexity of the concept of stress, it makes it extremely difficult, often unrealistic and unsuitable, to identify stress 100% accurately. Instead, it is much more appropriate to explore a range of concerns which may lead to a person's appraisal of stress, i.e. his/her individual dimensions of stress. It is essential for the cancer nurse to adopt an individualistic approach, reflective of the transactional model of stress (see Chapter 1).

When cancer nurses make assumptions about anxiety and its intensity, they are not carrying out an effective assessment. Welch McCaffrey emphasises that cancer nurses must always be wary of making judgements based on assumptions, rather than deliberative assessments. She identifies the following categories of assessment which will help the nurse to identify anxiety in individual persons.

General variables eliciting anxiety

Ask the person to complete the sentence, **'I feel most anxious when...'** (Each of us may cite specific situations that tend to increase our anxiety threshold.)

Behavioural symptoms

An important component of an anxiety response is the behavioural characteristics of such. Ask the person, 'How would I know when you're anxious?' 'Do you act differently or exhibit certain behavioural **cues?'** (These are examples of open-ended questions which encourage the person to ventilate his/her feelings.)

Coping strategies

It is important to determine the person's customary response to a crisis situation. Much of what we can anticipate in coping with the cancer experience will be similar to how the person has coped with past stressful situations. Questions to ask the person include, **'How do you deal with uncertainty?'** and **'How have you coped with past crises?'**

Current stressors

It cannot be assumed that anxiety is elicited by the same factors in all persons. Therefore, an individualised approach to assessing causes of anxiety would integrate the question, **'What factors are potentiating anxiety now?'** This is a crucial question for effective intervention planning.

These categories are very specific and do not include all aspects of stress (as outlined by Lazarus, 1966). However, they are useful as main categories to which others can be added. It is important to note that the broader concept 'stress' can be inserted in the place of the stress emotion 'anxiety', in order to give a wider perspective.

Assessment creates the groundwork for the next stage of the nursing process, i.e. intervention planning. McCaffrey argues that intervention planning is based in part in the answer to the query, **'What worries you the most right now?'** Thus, there is a natural progression which involves monitoring a person's problems.

Patient education

A key nursing issue for the last few years has been that of patient education. As nurses have a significant amount of contact with patients, they constitute the 'front-line psychological workers' to provide teaching and support (Nichols, 1985). The nurse needs to act as the central resource person and can guide clients in exploring their environment, helping to reduce stress so that the clients may live lives that are meaningful for them. Health education forms one of the most essential functions of the nurse, however, it is still poorly understood and greatly undervalued (Poletti, 1984; Webb, 1988).

Welch McCaffrey (1984) notes that anxiety in the cancer experience is often related to a misunderstanding about the illness of cancer and/or its treatment. Educating patients plays an important role in anxiety reduction. However, she acknowledges that the recognition of individual preferences for the degree of information is important. There is no universal and finite amount of information that is required by persons with a diagnosis of cancer. Increased knowledge and understanding is often sought out by patients because it promotes a sense of control in their lives with a corresponding decrease in anxiety.

Methods of information-giving regarding the reduction of anxiety vary. Individual teaching may reduce anxiety and allow for an informal, personalised approach to teaching. Group options for teaching offer other alternatives. Elevated levels of anxiety decrease knowledge retention, hence, reinforcement of information is crucial and the timing of teaching may predict the degree of information retention (Welch McCaffrey, 1985).

Friedenbergs *et al* (1980) developed a programme consisting of educating the person regarding his/her disease and how to utilise supports to alleviate anxiety. The programme includes familial and environmental supports, educational materials describing the disease, relaxation techniques and *in vivo* emotive imagery (e.g. encouraging the person to think of pleasant thoughts, memories and events).

In the United States, careful planning of patient education is widely accepted and is considered to be of crucial importance in a person's effective progress. This is reflective of the current emphasis on cancer rehabilitation. Specific structured educational programmes which form an integral part of the nursing process are currently in use.

Cancer rehabilitation is a holistic approach aimed at improving the quality of life of a chronically ill person. The nurse employs the skills of assessment, teaching and counselling and actively involves the person with cancer and his/her family in the programme (Whelan, 1984; Johnson, 1980; Corkle, 1984; Turner, 1985).

Johnson devised a structured educational rehabilitation programme for a group of approximately fifty individuals with cancer, to measure its effects on their knowledge of specific aspects of their disease and its implications. The education sessions were carried out over a four week period and included specific goals and learning objectives (e.g. learning about the disease; coping with daily health problems; communicating with others; liking yourself; living with limitations and finding resources that can help). The individuals had access to a learning resource centre which had audio-visual aids. Johnson strongly suggested from her results that such a programme does significantly reduce the levels of anxiety of persons with cancer. It also increases their knowledge about their disease and gives a sense of meaning to their lives.

Fredette and Beattie (1986) developed a patient education programme in order to assist individuals with cancer to achieve and maintain an optimum state of health. They wished to provide

information, reduce anxiety, minimise the sense of hopelessness and foster hope. Thus, their programme does not cater solely for information needs, but also for psychosocial issues. Its focus lies with group sharing of thoughts, concerns, questions and suggestions. The programme includes the use of special videotapes covering common problems, which are then used to stimulate discussion amongst the group. Hence, teaching takes the form of a participative process. However, Fredette and Beattie ask how they can reach people who want and need information but do not feel comfortable attending this structured programme. The answer to their question may lie in a much more informal, individual approach. It can be seen that many American assessment schedules and education programmes that have been developed over the last ten years are highly structured, formal and group oriented. There clearly needs to be development in assessment and programmes aimed directly at the individual level of the person with cancer, in order to respond effectively to his/her support needs.

As Hitch and Murgatroyd (1985) recommend, there should be more information regarding psychosocial aspects of care. They suggest that such information should be recorded routinely in the case notes. A study found that, where forms to record information about diagnosis and related issues had been incorporated in a person's notes, communication improved. Thus, by incorporating this information, continuity of communication over a span of time should be ensured (Lyal, 1984).

Conclusion

It can be seen that many individuals develop largely negative attitudes towards cancer. Hence, there are conceptual links with Lazarus' model of stress (1966) (see Chapter 1), as many individuals are likely to appraise cancer as a threat and, subsequently, experience stress. It is worth noting that the diverse range of concerns outlined by health care literature reveals individual variations in the causes of stress for the person with cancer. These concerns can be further usefully explored with reference to relevant psychological theory. This helps to substantiate the research and create a holistic picture of stress as applied to the person with cancer.

5   Psychological concepts pertaining to stress and persons with cancer

Perceptions of illness and health

It is important to study perceptions of illness and health, as an individual's perceptions of these will influence how stress is appraised when faced with a life-threatening chronic illness. If stress is appraised, perceptions of illness and health will also affect the nature and degree of stress experienced and, subsequently, help to determine ways of coping with the illness. Thus, a psychological analysis of perceptions of the constructs of health and illness is essential in order to gain an holistic understanding of the concept of stress, as applied to individuals with cancer. This chapter includes an overall view of people's fundamental ideas relating to the broad concepts of health and illness. To conclude, there is an exploration of the key factors influencing individuals' perceptions of health and illness which consequently affect their behaviour.

Concepts of health and illness

Herzlich (1973) provides a comprehensive psychosociological discussion of persons' perceptions of health and illness from in-depth unstructured interviews. Her account begins with a historical overview of deep-seated theories relating to the genesis of illness and the origins of health. Historians of medicine commonly put forward two causal concepts of illness:

- The view that illness is endogenous. Illness is represented by the individual who plays a major part in its genesis.
- The view that illness is exogenous. Illness is due to noxious elements in the earth, hence the way of life of each person is important.

Today, many individuals tend to equate the urban way of life, in particular, with illness. They possess an exogenous view of illness. A respondent in Herzlich's study vividly explains how an urban way of life is synonymous with diseases of modern life (in this case cancer), which, for many respondents, represented the most significant picture of illness:

Cancer I rather associate with current allergies, with very modern allergic diseases, with the physical and nervous strain we undergo in cities and then in breathing in present day atmosphere in cities.

However, an endogenous view of illness continues to play a role in today's society, i.e. that the individual does play a part in the genesis of illness and health. Each person has a variable capacity for resistance to disease. This partly depends on a complex interplay of a diverse range of physical and psychosocial factors, e.g. an individual's predisposition towards illness, personality, perceptions of illness and health (Herzlich, 1973). This view parallels Lazarus' transactional model of stress, as the key concept is the interaction between the individual and his/her environment.

Persons' perceptions of health

The definition of health is extremely difficult to analyse because health is a relative and **not** an absolute concept. It depends on subjective interpretation. Herzlich developed three broad themes regarding perceptions of health:

- 'Not being ill', i.e. an absence of illness. This represents a negative view of health, as the individual does not actually think of his/her health, or notice it, until it is lost. There is a general lack of awareness of one's body. However, if a historical view of health is taken, it is not surprising to find that health would be viewed in this way, because disease, even in the late Victorian era, was a common occurrence (e.g. tuberculosis, bronchitis, pneumonia and cholera were 'killer' diseases, Osborne, 1968).

- Health as a capital asset, i.e. an individual has good health because of their reserve of health. This is based on his/her physical robustness and psychological resistance to illness. Today, it can be seen that more persons are increasingly viewing health as a measure of physical fitness. Physical fitness includes the 'extra' energy needed to carry out everyday activities and have enough left over for any other activity (Hoffman, 1977). People, as a result of media coverage on healthy living, are becoming more aware of their bodies.

- An autonomous experience. The individual feels that he/she has equilibrium; everything is going well for them. This clearly links with a phenomenological approach (see Chapter 1), as it is rooted in the individual and their unique experiences. Herzlich labels this concept 'real' health, because it is a personal norm of life and it includes physical and psychological well-being.

This relates to Maslow's concept of self-actualisation (1957). Herzlich notes that this perception of health is referring to an optimum state **not** a perfect state.

She acknowledges that there exists, for many individuals, an intermediate state between health and illness which she refers to as generalised fatigue. There is also an increased liability to illness due to decreased personal resistance. The key element is the individual's perceptions of his/her physical or mental state. A state of being well can be viewed as a continuum, ranging from a sub-optimum level of barely being well to a high level of 'wellness' or optimum health.

Persons' perceptions of illness

Herzlich identified three **main** themes regarding perceptions of illness from her study:

- Illness as destructive. This theme corresponds with those respondents who are active in society. For these individuals, illness tends to be equated with desocialisation and individual solitude. They view health as being synonymous with the social world. Illness is the total opposite, a loss of social role. Illness is seen as deviance and is regarded as a negative influence because it often leads to dependence on others. The behaviour of these individuals at different stages may vary from complete rejection of the illness to complete passivity, when they are finally overcome by the illness.

- Illness as a liberator. For some individuals, illness is seen as a break away from social constraints, 'the blotting out of everyday'. In this way, illness becomes almost a pleasant experience, as it gives an individual time and is viewed as rest. It is more likely to be adopted by individuals with benign, short-lived illnesses (e.g. a common cold) (Kent and Dalgleish, 1983). In comparison, for individuals with cancer, their illness is much more likely to be appraised as a stressful experience due to the nature of the illness (see p76 on stigma).

    However, Herzlich also found that for a minority of persons with experience of a serious disease, illness was viewed as a desocialisation process, yet meant enrichment of the individual (e.g. possession of intellectual activities, power from the possession of certain privileges and a liberation of personality with a lifting of social constraints). The individual's personality may become much more positive, in that the person develops an increased sensitivity towards other people. The individual may also become more reflective and aware of him/herself as a person. It is more likely that this positive reaction to cancer occurs when an individual is in remission and is able to maintain optimum quality of life.

- Illness as an occupation. The function of the person is to fight the illness, the sole aim being to get better. The individual needs energy to undertake this and is given by release from the roles of everyday life. The individual does not have the time for other roles. Herzlich gives an example of a woman with cancer who explains:

> *Illness is an occupation... for me, it's more of an occupation when I can put up a fight against my illness. Now I no longer fight because I'm working, I haven't the time.*

For many persons with cancer who face a long period of intensive treatment and related physical illness, the disease is likely to be the main occupation. The key feature of this perception of illness is that the person sees illness as a period to get through. The individual is constrained to accept his/her illness (this shows the illness' power). However, the person has power, in the sense that he/she endures the illness and aims to overcome it. Herzlich explains that the person's relationship with the doctor is important, as the individual desires information, aims to be co-operative and participates in the treatment.

This theme closely parallels Parker's sociological analysis (1985) of the change process in persons with leukaemia, which he labels the 'cancer passage'. There are similar role demands, as the average requirements of the patient's role, which constitute the external dimension of cancer passage, are shaped to a large extent by a strongly medicalised system of meaning and action in high technology, hospital-based care (Parker, 1985).

Yet this third theme is too simplistic, as the process of becoming ill is **not** synonymous with the adoption of the patient role. Herzlich's descriptions, regarding illness as destructive and as a liberator, illustrate this point. In contrast to Parson's (1951) functional approach, Mechanic (1968) views 'illness behaviour' as being a complex issue; something that is not always morally neutral. He explains that sickness can be seen as deviant behaviour. Herzlich's description of illness as destructive is clearly applicable here, e.g. lung cancer is often linked with heavy smoking; cancer of the cervix with promiscuity. The stigma attached to these illnesses may have an effect on a person's life, to the extent that he/she refuses to adopt the sick role (see p76 on stigma).

Mechanic adopts a phenomenological approach, as he emphasises that symptoms are differentially perceived, evaluated and acted upon by different kinds of people and in different situations. The decision as to whether to consult a doctor is complex and depends on many variables, e.g. the extent of the disruption of everyday activities, situational factors and the frequency and persistence of symptoms. The individual with an illness does not decide whether to adopt the role of patient in isolation, as he/she usually discusses it with significant others. Friedson (1968) refers to this as the 'lay referral system'. Persons are influenced in their concept of self by the reaction of others. The sick role may or may not become part of the person's self-image. Relinquishing the sick role is **not** synonymous with physiological recovery from a condition. The individual may not automatically return to his/her previous state of activity. Recovery from illness is only indirectly related to an objective state of health (Kent and Dalgleish, 1983).

In more widespread terms, there are also significant transcultural factors to consider. Zola (1966) discovered that in different cultures some symptoms of illness are more important than others. He puts forward the hypothesis that, if the prevalence of a symptom in the population is more widespread, it is more likely that the community will regard it as normal. He also proposes the hypothesis of the congruence of a symptom with a society's dominant value orientations, i.e. how the symptom fits/misfits with mainstream norms and values. Zola argues that there are clear cultural differences which influence an individual's decision-making to become a patient.

Conclusion

To conclude, Herzlich's (1973) analysis of persons' perceptions of health and illness acts as a useful framework for a study of the key dimensions involved. A phenomenological approach, as adopted in this text, allows for the realisation of the diversity of individual influences affecting the overall perceptions of illness and health. This, in turn, enables a fuller understanding of the complex meanings of stress and coping in relation to individuals with cancer.

6   Concept of pain

Introduction to concept of pain

The concept of pain links to the transactional model of stress, as the individual is likely to appraise the experience of pain as a harmful event. Thus, perceptions of stress often ensue. Indeed, stress may also intensify the individual's experience of pain, due to the relationship between mood states within the higher centre of the brain and pain impulses. This chapter aims to explore the concept of pain to further understand its links with stress and the person with cancer. The following aspects are considered:

- outline of the physiological and psychosocial aspects of pain;
- cancer pain and its dimensions;
- pain assessment.

Outline of physiological and psychosocial aspects of pain

Melzack and Wall's gate control theory (1982) contributes to a more comprehensive view of pain, as they acknowledge the multidimensional properties of pain experience and behaviour. The gate lies within the spinal cord and, in certain circumstance, it allows nerve impulses from pain stimulation to pass through and be felt. When the gate is open, pain impulses flow through. However, when it is closed, none pass through and pain is not experienced. The degree of opening is influenced by connections within the central nervous system. It takes into account the higher centres of the nervous system. Here, an evaluation of input takes place and past experience plays an important part, i.e. it exerts control over the sensory-discriminative aspect of pain (signal of tissue damage). It also influences the activities within the reticular and limbic structures which account for motivational drive and possible unpleasant, affective characteristics.

This theory offers a conceptual framework for the integration of sensory, emotional and behavioural dimensions of pain. The inclusion of the influence of higher centres within the brain and the role of past experience gives support to the argument that pain is a highly qualitative concept, which is individualistic and subject to change. Pain differs from person to person and culture to culture (Melzack and Wall, 1984; Sofaer, 1984). McCaffrey (1983) explains that pain is what the patient says it is and exists when he says it does. Similarly, Bonica (1979) perceives pain to be a subjective, personal experience that cannot be seen, touched or measured.

Psychogenic pain

It follows that an individual's pain experience is influenced by the person's unique personal history, state of mind and the meaning attached to pain. A sound knowledge of psychological factors influencing pain is helpful in order to understand a person's reactions to his/her pain experience.

Merske and Spear (1967) suggested that a complaint of pain may equally constitute a symptom of a psychological, as well as a physiological, disorder. Their theory explores the links with anxiety and depression. Acute pain (of recent onset or short duration) is an emergency response, which is similar to an acute anxiety attack. When the person is given anti-anxiety drugs for acute pain, the pain decreases. A person's mental and physical states vary with time and this has a clear effect on the severity, tolerance and expression of pain. Hayward (1975) acknowledged that pain is influenced by anxiety. He hypothesised that anxiety is influenced by information about future events. His research revealed that giving relevant preoperative information reduced postoperative pain and anxiety.

Chronic pain has been defined as pain of at least several months' duration. If the pain is constant, there develops an habituation of the amount of response within the central nervous system and 'vegetative signs' begin, e.g. sleep disturbance, appetite changes, decreased libido and increased irritability, which are also signs of depressive reactions (Sternbach, 1978). In psychosocial terms, the individual's life is severely altered by chronic pain, to such an extent that the person may be unable to function socially and may experience difficulty with other activities of daily living. Depression often occurs as a result of the person's situation. If the person is treated for depression, the pain is likely to be reduced.

Psychosocial aspects influencing the experience of pain range from early life experiences; the present environment; the meaning an individual attaches to pain and his/her cultural background. These factors give rise to personal attitudes of pain which influence pain expression. As pain is a complex experience, influenced by diverse factors, nurses should adopt an holistic approach (i.e. one which encompasses biological, psychological and sociocultural factors) in order to deal with all aspects of a person's pain (Waugh, 1988).

Cultural influences

Pain thresholds vary little from one person to another; the difference lies in an individual's communication patterns concerning his/her pain. A study of ethnic groups in America found that both inhibited the expression of pain, but for different reasons. The Old Americans tended to 'take it in their stride'. The Irish Americans were afraid to appear 'like babies'. In contrast, two other groups encouraged pain expression but for different reasons. The Italian Americans rallied support, expected, and were satisfied with, relief from the pain. The Jewish Americans valued catharsis, as it brought attention to the possible cause of pain (Zborowski, 1969).

As it is impossible for nurses to directly feel a person's suffering, they have to rely on their own judgements and inferences. This gives rise to the function of personal systems of beliefs regarding suffering. These include stereotypes of people belonging to various cultural backgrounds. A study revealed that the ethnic or religious background of a patient proved to be a significant determinant of the nurse's inference of the individual's suffering. The American nurses in the study by Davitz and Davitz (1981) believed that Jewish and Spanish patients suffered most, while Oriental and Anglo-Saxon Germanic patients suffered least.

Cross-cultural differences among nurses were also reported in the study by Davitz and Davitz. For example, for Nepalese and Chinese nurses, psychological motivation is not part of their cultures and, when working in America, these nurses were surprised by the turmoil experienced by American persons regarding illness. In contrast, Puerto Rican nurses rated more psychological distress as opposed to physiological pain. Davitz and Davitz's study highlights the importance of one's belief systems in the assessment of pain and the need to recognise this in order to prevent cultural bias.

Cancer pain and it dimensions

Psychosocial factors also play a central role in the experience of cancer pain. The problem of cancer pain is significant due to its prevalence and intensity. For many persons with recurrent cancer, pain develops and often becomes increasingly severe. This causes both a physiological and psychological deterioration in their general condition. A third of persons experience moderate to severe pain in the intermediate stage of cancer and this rises to 60-80% for persons with advanced disease (Bonica, 1990). For persons admitted to a provincial hospice, 58% experienced pain as their major symptom (Wilkes, 1979). These figures are clear illustrations of the significance of the experience of pain for the person with advanced cancer. It is likely that, for these individuals, stress forms a part of their everyday lives. It has been argued that malignant disease causes total pain, as it constitutes a combination of physical, emotional and spiritual suffering (Saunders, 1984).

Due to its prevalence and intensity, cancer pain has a greater physiological and psychological impact than a non-malignant illness on the person. As in chronic pain, the person with severe cancer pain is likely to experience physiological deterioration, e.g. lack of sleep, reduced appetite, nausea and vomiting. This, in turn, leads to psychological effects as the person is likely to become depressed and experience feelings of helplessness. If pain therapy fails, the individual may become increasingly bitter and more preoccupied with the pain, losing interest in his/her social activities. Pain becomes the central focus and dominates the person's life (Bonica, 1990).

Fear of pain is often second only to fear of death. Both death and pain are universal human experiences. Nurses begin to recognise and avoid persons who are dying, as it is often a painful realisation of their own vulnerability. Equally, this could be the reason why nurses avoid persons with pain and sometimes deny or doubt their pain. McCaffrey (1983) asks if we are trying to quieten our terror and avoid facing our vulnerability to pain.

Responses of fear, resentment, anger and anxiety at the diagnosis and prognosis of cancer, all enter into the experience of pain and contribute to pain behaviour. For example, many individuals experience intense fear with any ache or pain, as it could possibly be a symptom of the disease spreading (Chapman, 1979).

If a person's significant others do not share the same pain-related attitudes and behaviours, this may lead to communication difficulties and resulting isolation for the person. Often, persons do not like to discuss their pain with others, or are ambivalent about it. Persons with cancer are especially aware of the social stigma attached to complaining about pain (McCaffrey, 1983). Problems of communication about pain between nursing staff and patients may occur. For example, the individual may expect the staff to know all about his/her pain, as it is 'typical' for them, and, hence, presume it needs no explaining. Yet, equally, the staff may rely on the person to tell them about his/her pain (Raiman, 1988).

There are also the wide implications of role change within a family unit. Pain and illness often interfere with role function. McCaffrey also acknowledges the effect of the emotions anxiety, fear and depression (elicited by the cancer pain) on relationships. These emotions tend to heighten the person's interpretation of situations and creates a highly emotional climate. McCaffrey explores the fight between dependence and independence for persons with cancer — some struggle on with the pain, while others accept the help of the family but do not perceive their strain. She concludes that many factors related to cancer pain may hamper the person's relations with others.

The family provides the context in which the pain occurs. A study found that those spouses who were highly stressed, rated their partner's pain significantly higher than the group of less stressed spouses, even though the levels of pain as reported by persons with cancer in each group were almost identical. Over half the spouses in the study were experiencing some form of health disturbance, which they attributed to their partners' pain. The pain of a partner also clearly has a psychological effect, as spouses experience a sense of helplessness at being unable to effect any change in this pain. The nature of family contact with health care professionals becomes critical. When there are no immediate answers forthcoming with regard to pain, feelings of anger and frustration are often experienced by family members. Hence, the family, similar to the person with cancer, is faced with learning how to live with the pain (Rowat, 1985). Indeed, cancer pain may form the person's overriding concern, which affects all other aspects of his/her life, from everyday living to unfulfilled plans.

Pain assessment

It can be seen that pain is a highly complex concept. Therefore, it is not surprising that the assessment of pain requires a careful, systematic approach. How do we recognise cues regarding a person's pain? The so-called 'objective' signs, such as increased blood pressure, pulse and respiration rates, are not problem-free. The lack of objective signs does not necessarily equal lack of pain, as the person may have learnt to adapt to the pain (i.e. to exert increased self control). Likewise, the amount of tissue damage is not an accurate predictor of pain. Studies of war victims reveal that many men did not verbalise about their pain, despite extensive damage, because of socialisation patterns concerning masculinity and the ethos of the war hero.

If we recognise that the experience of pain is a highly subjective one, then verbal communication, as emphasised by Lazarus (1966), is likely to be seen as one of the most valid indicators of the pain experience of the individual. This is because it is the individual's own report of his/her experience of the pain. The individual is the expert with respect to the pain experience.

This premise lies at the basis of the work of Melzack and Torgerson (1971) and the development of the McGill Pain Questionnaire. Their work began by attempting to specify the qualities of the concept of pain. They attempted to explore different aspects of the pain experience by putting words into classes and subclasses. This led to the development of the following areas:

- Sensory qualities — temporal aspects (whether the pain is constant or intermittent; whether it is precipitated by position, actions, weather, throughout the day and night), spatial, pressure, thermal. Examples of adjectives: throbbing, burning.

- Affective qualities — emotional responses to pain, which can directly influence the severity of the pain experience, e.g. tension, fear and autonomic properties. Adjectives include: sickening, terrifying.

- Evaluative qualities — this relates to the subjective overall intensity of the pain experience. Adjectives include: annoying, miserable.

The person is able to choose the category that most accurately describes the pain at any given moment in time. It also includes an overall pain intensity called the 'Present Pain Intensity' (PPI). This is based on a six point ordinal scale ranging from mild discomfort to horrible and excruciating.

Melzack acknowledges that it is essential to assess the patient as a person. It is not an objective measure, but an attempt to explore the different aspects of a person's pain experience through the words individuals use to describe pain. The questionnaire has been shown to give reliable and valid indicators of pain, and to be sensitive to detect differences among different methods to relieve pain. It not only gives information regarding the nature of painful sensations, but also explores how the pain experience is affecting the person's life. It is comprehensive, as it fulfils the function of pain assessment outlined by McCaffrey (1983) (i.e. it involves communication with the person on the subject of pain; it classifies pain; it characterises the pain sensation; it explores the effects of pain on the person and examines the factors influencing the person's pain experience).

Other, more traditional, approaches to the assessment of pain include the simple descriptive scale, which includes the adjectives severe, moderate, mild and absent. Obviously, this is a crude form of measurement and does not allow for more subtle individual differences. A pain thermometer has been developed at Burford's Nursing Development Unit (Pearson, 1987), which expands upon these adjectives by making them more amenable to patient use: no pain at all, a little pain, quite a lot of pain, a very bad pain, as much pain as I could possibly bear. The nurse and patient decide how often the 'painometer' will be used and analgesia can then be administered accordingly. The pain diary has been developed at the Pain Relief Unit in London (Raiman, 1988). On each form of the diary, the person is asked to fill in a line indicating the severity or otherwise of his/her pain each day. Both these examples are useful to help nurses improve pain relief. However, they are limited in their use, as they serve to give an overall impression of pain intensity and exclude possible causative factors.

The visual analogue scales are used extensively in the assessment of pain, similar to the quality of life scales. The key advantages reported are their sensitivity and uniformity — there are equal numbers of measures at all points along the line. Visual analogue scales have been useful to establish the value of treatments in clinical trials (Huskisson, 1977; Melzack, 1983). However, problems include failure to understand the concept of pain. It is difficult for many individuals to complete the visual analogue scales, in spite of careful instructions and practice, hence reducing their validity. There is also variation in reproducibility along the length of the line and doubts regarding the relationship of the measurement to the true pain experience (Huskisson, 1977). This is a significant problem, as the visual analogue scales only yield estimates of a unidimensional character, i.e. pain intensity. The scales cannot explore the multidimensional properties of the pain experience. Thus, for an assessment of pain intensity and its different qualities, the McGill Pain Questionnaire is more appropriate.

Other forms of assessment include graphic representations. These are useful to facilitate communication between the person and medical and nursing staff. The pain chart assesses the temporal aspects of pain, records the timing and intensity of the pain and circumstances associated with it. It is important that the charting of the pain is as close to the time of its occurrence as possible to prevent any potential bias. The pain chart, with regard to the spatial properties of pain, consists of a two-dimensional graphic account which reports the number of subjective components of the presenting pain problem. Hence, it relies upon the person to show exactly where all his/her pains are upon body charts (Huskisson, 1977). Raiman's (1986) London Hospital Pain Chart is a comprehensive example, as it records the location and severity of pain at regular intervals and the effect of the analgesia given. The chart aims to increase the communication between the person, nurse and doctor, making the recording of pain more systematic. It also makes useful information readily available in one place when taking decisions about pain management. Finally, it focuses attention on the mechanisms of different pains and it provides evidence on what relieves them, as it records each site of pain separately. Pain charts serve a specific purpose and are useful if used with other forms of assessment, so that all aspects of a person's pain experience are explored.

A pain profile and history, in conjunction with assessment methods, is essential. The profile consists of a series of straightforward questions which help to establish facts about the pain, including: time, past, present, duration, variation, location, nature, relief, coping, effect activities, emotion and treatment (Raiman, 1988).

A study revealed that nurses failed to record key aspects of a person's pain (i.e. location, quality, pattern, intensity, factors associated with pain, verbal statements, non-verbal expression and symptoms associated with pain). The nurses recorded approximately two of the eight categories and less than half of the person's perceptions of pain information was documented (Camp, 1988). Inadequate documentation regarding pain factors is common and there remains a lack of knowledge regarding pain assessment and the documentation process (Fox, 1982).

Conclusion

To conclude, pain is a highly qualitative experience which encompasses a wealth of physiological and psychosocial factors. Lazarus' transactional model of stress is highly appropriate because, similar to the concept of stress, the individual's perceptions of pain experience are of central concern. Assessment of an individual's pain which focuses on his/her verbal reports is much more likely to reflect the pain experience as it is actually perceived by the individual.

7 Concept of helplessness

This chapter aims to examine the concept of helplessness in order to further explore the effects of the perceived lack of control outlined by Lazarus (see Chapter 1, p8).

The phenomenon of helplessness and its association with ill health has been extensively studied by Seligman. He defines helplessness as a psychological state which frequently develops when events are **perceived to be** uncontrollable, i.e. when whatever form of action the subject takes makes no difference to the outcome of events, or when nothing can be done to influence an outcome.

In his first animal experiment with a dog and a shuttlebox, the dog is potentially subject to shocks, which it can escape by jumping over a barrier when it hears a tone which precedes the shock. In normal circumstances, the dog quickly learns to avoid the shock. Yet, dogs who have undergone classical conditioning appear to 'give up' and lay on the floor, whimpering. They accept the shocks passively, without seeking to escape. He concluded that when an organism experiences trauma it cannot control, the motivation to respond to other trauma is reduced, even when the organism responds and the response brings relief. The organism still has trouble learning that the response works.

Seligman discusses the relevance of learning theory. Only when an organism has learned by experience that an event is uncontrollable does it lead to helplessness. At first, the organism is able to cope with the event and uses all known or available methods to control the situation. When these are no longer available, real exhaustion sets in with the realisation that the situation is uncontrollable. This frequently leads to feelings of helplessness, which, for humans, presents as illness in the form of depression and anxiety.

This explanation resembles the GAS reaction syndrome of Selye (1957), as it is a macro-explanation of human behaviour which does not take human variation into account. Also similar to Selye's work, is Seligman's finding that continued exposure to the stimulus (e.g. failure at work, death of a loved one or newly diagnosed cancer) leads to a chronic situation, and even death, for the person. The depressed person believes that he/she cannot control those elements of life that relieve suffering. The person feels helpless. This may ultimately lead to premature death. Again, this is a generalisation of human occurrences and, therefore, fails to take into account the varying experiences of individuals.

It has been argued that, with humans, susceptibility to helplessness is determined by **perceived** control rather than actual control (Glass and Singer, 1972). For example, consider a person being admitted to hospital. On admission, a hospital bed is allocated, a wrist label is attached and the nurses are allowed to take over responsibility and care, i.e. the individual adopts the patient role. If the person has not been in hospital before, he/she is placed in a situation, such as ward routine, that is alien to that person; one in which he/she **appears** to have little control. The person is in the hands of the professionals, who have the knowledge and power to treat the person. It is easy to see how, in this situation, a person's stress level rises and anxiety and depression may develop.

However. studies regarding the nature of the professional–patient relationship suggest that it forms a much more complex relationship. Not all patients are passive and this clearly links with Lazarus'phenomenological theory of stress, as he emphasises that the individual takes an active part in a situation and events do not simply happen. Thus, the individual does play a crucial part in the proceedings. Power exists on both sides of the doctor–patient relationship, although it is highly skewed in the doctor's favour. The distribution of power is related to the distribution of knowledge. The doctor is extremely powerful, as he/she possesses highly specialised medical knowledge. Yet, the person may have some knowledge regarding general notions of health and illness and the ability to subjectively determine what is usual or wrong, i.e. the individual knows his/her body better than anyone else. This leaves the person with some power. Hence, the person is not simply a passive being in which events simply happen (Tuckett, 1976; Dingwall, 1977).

Even though power differences exist, feelings of powerlessness (i.e. **no authority** to act, although the individual does not necessarily perceive him/herself to be helpless) can be avoided during the patient–professional interaction, via a process of negotiation. Albrecht (1971) defines successful negotiation as based upon a reciprocal relationship, good rapport, open communication, clear understanding of the issues and goal consensus. He accepts that each party has its own interests with respect to a situation. Their relationship, however, is symbiotic because neither party will achieve their goals without co-operation from the other party. Social exchange theory, or, in Goffman's terms (1967), 'trade-offs', means that exchanges usually result in a compromise acceptable to each party. These exchanges mean that the patient is less likely to believe that events are outside his/her control. This is directly in keeping with the humanistic notion of the individual as an active agent in given situations. It also reveals the complexity of the concept of helplessness as applied to human beings.

There are instances in the nurse–patient relationship when the patient uses his/her power to influence the situation. For example, the nurse may ask the person with cancer to perform a task, such as checking the treatment area during the course of radiotherapy, which the nurse perceives as helping towards a person's recovery. The person may refuse to do this, as it is inconvenient at that particular time. The power shifts. By the process of negotiation, the nurse and the person may agree that the task can be carried out at a later time, suitable to them both. The nurse still gets the person to do the task, but, as the person took part in the decision over when it was to be done, the person's perception of helplessness was avoided. It is clearly important for persons to participate in their care and for nurses to undertake patient teaching, in order that persons do not experience feelings of helplessness and hence, avoid subsequent appraisals of stress.

The negotiated arena helps to explain the professional–patient interaction. It has been likened to a game of chess, with implicit negotiations and silent bargains. Patients negotiate as laymen (e.g. on a psychiatric ward, a patient may negotiate for more privileges, such as bed allocation and length of stay in hospital) (Strauss, 1978). It is also referred to as game-playing. These 'games' occur all the time in hospitals, without disturbing, and perhaps even helping to maintain, the structural context in which one side is ultimately more powerful (Long, 1976).

Conclusion

Feelings of helplessness result from an unequal distribution of power in the patient–professional interaction. The patient has been identified as the party most likely to develop significant stress appraisals, due to his/her relatively powerless position. However, the state of helplessness is **not** inevitable. The critical factor is the individual's perceived control of the situation. Hence, helplessness and its associated problems may be avoided by patient participation and a process of negotiation, which allows the person to express his/her views and aim for a consensus of goals between the professional and the patient.

8 Altered body image, sexuality and stigma

Introduction — altered body image and sexuality

It is important to explore the effects of altered body image and sexuality on individuals with cancer, in order to gain a detailed picture of how these affect an individual undergoing treatment for cancer. The philosophy of Lazarus' transactional model of stress is highly relevant to this analysis, as he emphasises the central role of the individual's perception of threat in the ensuing stress experience. The ways in which an individual with cancer appraises his/her altered body image determines the role of stress and the subsequent coping processes.

Outline of the role of body image

Body image forms a central part of our self concept in Westernised society. Society places significance on having an attractive body, so body image becomes an essential part of everyday living for individuals. This results in pressure to comply with the image the mass media portray and consequently creates problems for those who feel that their body image is not what it should be. Thus, what is expected of individuals by others can have a profound psychological effect (Salter, 1988). Rogers' theory of self concept (1967) emphasises the influence of significant others in shaping a person's self concept. Body image can be conceptualised as a mental picture of one's own body; the way in which the body appears to the self (Wood, 1975). It constitutes the sum of conscious and unconscious attitudes an individual has towards his/her body. An individual with a high level of self-esteem has a much clearer understanding of self (Chilton, 1984).

As body image is a continuing entity, it is constantly changing. This leads to the consideration of altered body image.

Altered body image and persons with cancer

The individual who is considered to present a body image which differs from social norms, suffers from stigma. The person concerned is either avoided or offered sympathy (see p76 on stigma). The individual goes through a grieving process due to actual or perceived loss of previous body image. Similar to the bereavement process, the person may go backwards and forwards through various stages until accepting his/her altered body image. For persons with cancer, the kind of illness they have, and the kind of loss they have to face, represents an attack on their own identity (Salter, 1988).

Cancer causes significant physical and psychological changes. Physical symptoms (e.g pain, weight loss, nausea and anorexia) can cause the person with cancer to alter attitudes towards his/her body. The notion of cancer cells present in the body, outside of the person's control, 'eating the body away' and invading good cells, can cause much anxiety for the person due to self-loss (Blackmore, 1988b).

Surgery

In surgery, actual procedures can cause an altered body image. This stems from actual physiological changes in bodily function or perceived change. Reactions to mutilating surgery are bound to the degree of development of a person's body image. Variations include age, sex, personality, beliefs, values, expectations and socio-cultural background. The degree of preparation for change, the cause of the change and relationship with health care professionals are equally relevant (Blackmore, 1988b; Wassner, 1986). Adaptation requires a change in the person's value system so that physical characteristics are less important, and the effects of the disability are confined, so that it does not affect uninvolved areas (Donovan and Pierce, 1976).

Radiotherapy

In radiotherapy, some symptoms can cause loss of control over body actions and a change in bodily function. Some individuals are virtually incontinent due to the effects of radiotherapy to the lower abdominal region. This often creates a negative body image, as it is altered by the use of sheaths or pads and is associated with regression to childhood (Salter, 1988). It is not surprising that fears and anxieties (e.g. fears of being burned, becoming disfigured or becoming sterile) are common amongst individuals receiving radiotherapy (Blackmore, 1988a, 1988b). These all have a significant impact on a person's perception of body image and subsequent appraisals of stress.

Chemotherapy

In chemotherapy, the effects of bone marrow depression can alter body appearance and function, and also change body action. Alopecia (baldness) is psychologically distressing, depending on the degree of importance placed on hair by the person, and may cause negative changes in body image perception. People in Westernised society have notions of suitability and beauty associated with having the 'right' amount of body hair (which differs for men and women). The loss of hair can be devastating, as it reduces a person's sense of attractiveness. It also acts as an ever-present reminder of the person's illness. Even if the individual is able to accept the change, there is still a doubt whether the treatment will be successful (Webb, 1985; Salter, 1988).

A small-scale study explored body image for those persons with cancer with and without alopecia. The prediction that alopecia negatively affects body image was confirmed. It was also found that men with alopecia indicated a **lower** self-esteem than women with alopecia (Baxley *et al*, 1984). The literature alludes to the idea that men adjust to baldness better, as alopecia is often a naturally occurring change in men. However, these results do not parallel this assumption. Baxley *et al* conclude that their results have implications for nursing care (i.e. nurses must spend at least as much time assisting men to adjust to alopecia as women). It is often easy for nurses to think that, because they become accustomed to seeing a person bald, that the person has also become accustomed to this. Obviously, for some individuals this is not the case.

Testicular cancer

Most men with testicular cancer are at the age when they are forming sexual relationships and perhaps contemplating fatherhood, thus, the value placed on the appearance and function of the testicles is high. For those who have orchidectomy, body image is altered: the physical appearance is different due to an empty sac and scarring. There is also a functional loss, due to reduced sperm levels or testosterone levels. In some instances, functional loss also involves problems with erection (Blackmore, 1988). Clearly, changes in perception of sexuality are relevant and are linked with an altered body image.

Gynaecological cancer

For women with gynaecological cancer, there are likely to be problems with altered body image, as women (and society at large) place great value on the functional purpose of the uterus. Its removal is often seen by the woman as equalling loss of femininity. Obviously, sexuality and altered body image are interlinked here, as with testicular cancer. The loss of menstrual flow signifies the loss of a necessary and valuable function for good health, as it serves as periodic cleansing for the body (Blackmore, 1988b). Some women have intense fears, arising from the loss of their uterus, regarding the survival and stability of their family or marital system. This is often in addition to fears regarding their loss of attractiveness as a woman. Actual physical changes can cause sexual difficulties resulting from dryness of the vagina (Sewell and Edwards, 1980).

The stigma often associated with cervical cancer may lead to feelings of guilt. The woman may view the disease as punishment for 'sexual misdemeanours' in the past. This may also affect relationships with her partner (Salter, 1988, see also section on stigma, p76).

Breast cancer

The female breast is often regarded as symbol of intrinsic femininity and sexual desirability, in addition to maternal comfort and succour. It is central to many people's views about 'being a woman'. The threat of surgery to the breast is dependent not only upon cultural values, but also on the significance the breast holds for each individual (Tait, 1988). The meaning of breasts to the individual consists of a complex interaction of factors; societal views of the breast, past learning from parents and friends, present experience of family and friends and the individual woman's personal view (Rutherford, 1988). It is highly likely, therefore, that an alteration or loss of a breast gives rise to varying levels of stress, according to the individual. The woman may no longer feel sexually attractive to her partner. Her self-confidence in maintaining her style of dress, through which she expresses her sexuality, may also be undermined (Webb, 1985).

Cancer poses a double-edged threat because, in addition to removal of the breast, the woman also has a potentially life-threatening disease. She may feel threatened, as she knows that treatments for breast cancer are often unpleasant and may not be fully effective in producing remission or an increased quality of life

(Webb, 1985). Emotional suffering often outweighs physical pain, due to a sense of mutilation, loss of feelings of femininity and the fear of death (Jamison, 1978). A study revealed that women whose prime concern was breast loss rather than having cancer, were more likely to require psychiatric referral later (Devlen and Baum, 1987).

It is important to realise the impact of altered body image, to establish how much body image mattered prior to diagnosis. It has been reported that one in three women develop sexual problems following mastectomy and one in four develop clinical anxiety and depression within the year following surgery. As a result, assessments of a patient's morale and feelings about sexuality are essential (Tait *et al*, 1982).

A study of women with lumpectomy found that they felt threatened by the body image disturbance, yet they could not identify it, as the breast was intact (Rutherford, 1988). However, if the woman sees herself as suffering a loss, does it matter if the loss is only a segment of the breast? Although previous literature points to less psychological disturbance than persons with mastectomy, the body image of women with lumpectomy is still negatively affected.

Loss of a limb

Permanent changes in body image, such as loss of a limb, cause emotional stress, as it often results in the individual doubting his/her ability to continue with everyday roles. Salter (1988) explains that the feeling of being a 'part person' can rapidly produce a state of mind that will swallow a personality and destroy the ability to think in a positive manner.

The person with a limb deformity may see him/herself as abnormal and, subsequently, feel unwanted as a sexual partner. Also, the effects of being ill and having to rely on others for assistance with hygiene may be viewed as a gross curtailment of personal autonomy. Maintaining an appearance forms part of a person's body image and an expression of personality. The sick role itself may lead to a violation of individuality, sexuality and a lowered self-esteem (Webb, 1985).

The loss of a limb may also cause phantom limb sensations, when the individual continues to experience sensations of the body part that has been removed. The previous body image persists, and the individual has not yet adjusted to the loss and so distorts the meaning of the stimuli in order to deny the loss. This reveals how resistant body image is to the effects of mutilation. It portrays the strength of the psychological aspects of body image within the subconscious mind of the individual (Webb, 1985; Salter, 1988).

Stoma

The formation of a stoma involves the anal-equivalent being placed on the abdomen in a prominent position. A stoma demands frequent attention and can, as a result, become a dominant part of the person's daily life. It is important to establish whether the person is fearful of people 'discovering the secret', as some people may go to great lengths to conceal their changed image (Salter, 1988). This has clear links with the concept of stigma. A stoma is a perfect agent with which to alienate a person from social activity, to encourage him/her to become a recluse and to create depression. The person can feel stigmatised by their family, friends of employer(s). This is due to the fact that incontinence is socially unacceptable and people react with shock and disgust at a stoma. It is not simply the appearance of the stoma (red, swollen and messy), but also the connotations associated with it; the violations it brings. It is not surprising that it reverses the healthy body image people usually have of themselves. There are also the sexual connotations associated with having a stoma. The person concerned now has an orifice which differs from a normal one. Some women may regard it as a phallic symbol. Men may regard themselves as having female characteristics as it may bleed when cleaned, likening it to menstruation (Salter, 1988).

For adaptation to the altered body image to occur, it is essential that the person accepts the appearance of the site of the alteration, is able to touch and explore it and can learn to care for it independent of the help of others. If this fails to occur, the individual will be unable to reintegrate his/her new body image. It often requires significant coping abilities on the part of the individual to accommodate the new body image (Donovan and Pierce, 1976).

Conclusion — altered body image

A humanistic approach, highlighted by Lazarus' transactional model of stress (see Chapter 1), allows for an exploration of an individual's perceptions regarding body image. It can be seen from the literature that, for many persons with cancer, an altered body image is probable. As a result, stress appraisals are common and individuals require much psychological support in order to develop a positive self image.

Outline of the concept of sexuality

Defining sexuality is not simple because, similar to pain, it is a vague concept and, although everyone knows what it is, no-one can really describe it. Freud (1924) explained that including everything connected with the differences between the two sexes in the definition is perhaps the only way of hitting the mark, but that this explanation is too general and imprecise.

The Sex Information and Education Council of the States (Lion, 1982) provides a comprehensive definition, stating that it refers to the totality of a person. It includes all of the aspects of the human being that relate specifically to being a boy or a girl, a woman or a man, and it is an entity subject to life-long dynamic change. The Council argues that sexuality reflects our human character, not solely our genital nature. It is concerned with the biological, psychological, sociological, spiritual and cultural variables of life, which by their effects on personality, determine interpersonal relations.

This reveals the importance of sexuality and aptly relates the concept within a humanistic framework, because sexuality is clearly a human attribute. Sexuality is one of the most basic human needs which is intrinsic to a person's whole being. It is concerned with the concept of ourselves as men and women (i.e. our manliness or femininity) as we see ourselves or as we would like to be. Sexuality concerns our fears and fantasies about ourselves and others. The definition also places sexuality within a holistic perspective, because it does not simply refer to the genital areas or to the sexual act, but affects all aspects of our being. It also acknowledges that sexuality is a constant phenomenon, as it is directly linked to our personality and the way in which we develop relationships with others. Sexuality cannot be switched on or off, because we are sexual beings all the time. It is also the recognition that sexuality, similar to our personality, is a dynamic phenomenon which is changing in expression all of the time (Glover, 1985; Blackmore, 1988).

Sexuality and persons with cancer

Given the prevalent negative attitudes surrounding cancer, it is difficult at times to view the person with cancer as a sexual being. The words 'sexuality' and 'cancer' may seem inappropriate to utter in the same breath, because 'sexuality' evokes images of love, life and beauty, whilst 'cancer' strikes fear and revulsion into the hearts of many individuals (Von Eschenbach and Shover, 1984) (see p24 on attitudes). Studies emphasise that, for the person with cancer, sexual involvement can give the person a sense of 'being alive' and can also offer warmth and comfort at a time when the person most needs it (Jones, 1984). It has been argued that sexual intimacy is one of the most rewarding and sought after experiences life has to offer, and its importance is not diminished by the experience of developing cancer (Derogatis and Kourtesis, 1981).

The reactions of relatives of a person with cancer can have a profound effect on the person's sexuality. For example, rejection due to fear of contagion or revulsion over physical changes, withdrawal and alienation from the individual with cancer, may all result in the individual experiencing emotions of anxiety, uncertainty and insecurity, as well as the pervasive frustration of being helpless (Blackmore, 1988). Negative moods, such as depression, are likely to dampen other emotional responses, including sexual libido, as the individual may feel unattractive. In the case of severe illness resulting in permanent handicap, there are likely to be profound implications sexually, as the individual and partner have to find new ways of expressing sexuality or accept that sexual activity can never be possible. This can take a significant period of adjustment (Webb, 1985).

Living with cancer may actually enhance some aspects of one's sexuality, because **confronting** cancer can enable some individuals to assess their lifestyle and relationship (Ainslie, 1984). For those already experiencing sexual conflict, it may provide them with a socially acceptable excuse 'for withdrawing from sexual activity (Golden, 1983). This example emphasises the importance of treating each person with cancer as an individual and not presuming that, for every person with cancer, the diagnosis has a detrimental effect upon his/her sexuality.

Cancer nurses' views of sexuality

Cancer nurses need to change their views of sexuality from a problem identification approach to a health promotion approach. They need to ask themselves how they would **promote** sexual health in persons with cancer. This represents an important shift in focus and links to the concept of sexuality as a central aspect of our whole being (Blackmore, 1988). This change in emphasis, however, depends on whether the cancer nurse feels comfortable to carry out the role. Too often, nurses have inadequate knowledge, understanding and comfort with their own sexuality and that of the person, which precludes them from fulfilling this role. The unwillingness or difficulty experienced by the person and the nurse in broaching the subject of sexuality occurs because it is still considered, to a large extend, a taboo topic. A conspiracy of silence often ensues.

Many individuals with cancer and their partners do have questions and sexual concerns they would like to discuss. However, they do not usually initiate the subject of sex, as they feel the staff are too busy and are reluctant to bother them with concerns about the effects of treatment on sexual function. Due to the diagnosis of cancer being a serious matter, the person may think they should be grateful 'just to be alive'. The individual may interpret the staff's silence about sexual concerns to mean his/her sex life is over. Thus, if a person does initiate a discussion of sexual consequences, it usually means that the situation is of major concern (Glover, 1985; Hogan, 1980; Smith, 1989).

Emotional reactions may occur when the person feels sexually threatened (as a result of illness). This may result in sexual joking and unwanted touching, in order to deny that the person's sexuality is threatened; or attempts to overcompensate for feelings of inadequacy by emphasising his masculinity/her femininity. These actions may provoke negative responses from staff (e.g. ignoring the person (see parallels with Stockwell's study, 1980 discussed on p15), yet these actions may form the person's only link with sexuality whilst in hospital. During and after illness, there is an increased need for the person to feel reassured that he/she can still receive and give sexual pleasure. This is difficult to communicate in hospital, where circumstances offer the individual little or no chance to express sexuality. The lack of provision of privacy to express emotions also reflects failure to respect the person's sexuality (Webb, 1985).

An American study of registered cancer nurses found that only 40% of staff identified discussion of sexual consequences as their responsibility (Camp, 1989). Often, the problem lies in discomfort in discussing the subject and the lack of formal education in personal attitudes regarding sexuality. Another study found that, by increasing the nurses' knowledge of sexuality, their attitudes became more accepting and, as a result, they were more comfortable in dealing with sexual issues (Fisher and Lewin, 1983). In order for the nurse to intervene and assist the person with cancer to maintain, attain or regain sexual health, the first requirement is education in sexuality, in conjunction with the use of supportive, non-judgmental communication techniques.

Cancer nurses should include sexual consequences of treatment as part of the information they provide to persons with cancer, giving individuals the opportunity to discuss concerns regarding sexuality and have their questions answered. Camp (1988) argues that it does not have to take a great deal of time, as frequently all that is necessary is a conversation which provides accurate information and helps the person accept his/her feelings towards cancer and sexuality.

Conclusion

To conclude, the concept of sexuality forms an integral part of a person's being and is a dynamic phenomenon. Lazarus' transactional model of stress provides an appropriate humanistic framework in which to explore the effects of cancer upon an individual's perception of his/her body image and sexuality.

The concept of stigma

Discussion of theory of stigma

The work of Goffman (1963) on stigma is highly relevant and contributes to a deeper understanding of this complex concept, in keeping with a humanistic perspective. Goffman's work focuses on persons with mental illness. However, parallels can be drawn with persons with cancer. Similar to the person with mental illness, the person with cancer possesses a trait (i.e. a diagnosis of cancer, as compared with a diagnosis of mental illness). Goffman explains that the trait can draw immediate attention and turn people the person meets away, because of his/her 'undesired differentness'.

The person with cancer, similar to the person with mental illness, may also experience shame due to the reaction of others. The individual perceives his/her own attributes (i.e. having cancer or mental illness) as being a defiling thing to possess. As regards the person with cancer, this view is more likely to be held by older generations of people for whom cancer was often viewed as a dirty or unclean disease to possess. For some individuals, cancer evokes powerful feelings of disgust and revulsion because it is seen as an unhygienic disease. Due to the profound ignorance which still surrounds the possible modes of transmission of the disease, beliefs founded on contagion are evident. A study found that some individuals no longer ate foods cooked by a person with cancer, nor drank from utensils used by a person with cancer and/or avoided direct physical contact (Fallowfield, 1988).

Normals (i.e. those people free from stigma) often act by exercising discrimination towards the stigmatised person, which often results in reduced life chances (Goffman, 1963). It can be seen that some persons with cancer have problems securing or maintaining a job, even when they are in remission from the illness and are physically capable of returning to work. The person with cancer may also find it difficult to resume family and social roles after a period of hospitalisation. This is likely to be due to significant others feeling that the person has a life-threatening illness and is expected to continue to adopt the sick role.

Goffman notes that the individual can attempt to correct his/her condition by devoting private effort to the mastery of areas felt to be closed on incidental and physical grounds. For example, some persons with cancer devote a significant proportion of their personal time when at home to fundraising activities for cancer research bodies. These may include active sporting events which require physical aptitude.

However, Goffman argues that it is also possible for the individual to use his/her stigma for secondary gains, i.e. as an excuse for the failure that has come their way. The person may use the stigmatised trait as a prop. For example, in some cases, persons with cancer may view their illness as being solely responsible for their unemployment, the failure of their marriage, the failure to secure close friends or failure to pass exams.

Yet, Goffman is careful to include a positive aspect associated with being stigmatised. He explains that the individual may see the trials suffered as a blessing in disguise. In other words, the notion that suffering can teach us about life and people. Sometimes, persons with cancer may comment that they feel they are 'better' people because they have learned to appreciate the important things in life (e.g. family). They may also comment that they are able to take each day at a time and live their life to the full. For example, some persons with cancer carry out unfulfilled dreams by travelling abroad or taking up a new hobby, whilst others relearn the simple pleasures of a warm summer's day.

When the stigmatised person meets other people in a social context, he/she does not know what the others are really thinking and often feels self-conscious about the impression made upon them. Goffman states that the individual's minor accomplishments may be assessed as signs of remarkable capacities. Yet, minor failings may be interpreted as a direct expression of the individual's stigmatised differentness, especially when that differentness can be perceived. As a result, people tend to stare and have a morbid curiosity about the stigmatised person's condition. Clearly, this applies to the person with cancer, whose appearance may be altered as a result of treatment (e.g. hair loss due to chemotherapy). The individual may feel extremely self-conscious and strangers may address him/her and start a conversation about the person's illness and treatment. The individual's friends, whilst commending his/her ability to get through the treatment, may also perceive other aspects of the person, such as a lack of social skills, as resulting solely from the illness.

Goffman notes that sympathetic others are often found who are ready to adopt the individual's standpoint and who will share the individual's stigma. These 'others' can provide the individual with instruction in the 'tricks of the trade' and can make him/her feel 'at home'. It can be seen that some individuals with cancer develop strong friendships with fellow patients whilst in hospital. The person is more inclined to accept other patients' information regarding treatment because they have actually gone through a similar course of treatment. This may not always prove a positive experience, however, as Goffman reports that fellow patients may focus on tales of atrocity. The person with cancer is likely to hear popular myths relating to the treatment, which may cause significant anxiety.

Group formation for stigmatised individuals, in the form of self-help groups, is discussed by Goffman. There are a diverse range of self-help groups for persons with cancer, relating to different sites of cancer (e.g. breast cancer support groups), in addition to national information and support agencies, such as BACUP and Cancer Link.

Goffman explains that at self-help groups exemplary moral tales are often provided which illustrate a desirable code of conduct. For example, persons with cancer may be told of a person who fought the illness courageously over a long period of time.

In addition to peer group support, Goffman explains that the individual can expect support from what he calls 'wise' normals who, due their special situation, are privy to the secret life of the stigmatised individual and sympathetic with it. The first type of 'wise' persons are those working in an establishment which caters to the needs of the individual with cancer. Goffman cites nurses as an example. With respect to the person with cancer, cancer nurses play a central role in the support for the individual and in the support for the person's family. The second type of 'wise' persons are the family members related to the stigmatised individual, who often share some of the discredit of being stigmatised (e.g. the spouse of the person with cancer may experience the distancing tactics of neighbours and friends).

The moral career of the stigmatised individual, in which an analysis of key stages in the individual's life takes place, is explored by Goffman. Initially, the stigmatised individual learns the standpoint of normals, and has a general idea of what it would be like to possess a particular stigma. Similarly, the person with cancer, prior to learning the nature of his/her illness, is likely to have general notions regarding cancer. In the second stage, the individual learns that he/she possesses a particular stigma and discovers the consequences of this in detail. The person with cancer, on learning the diagnosis, is given the implications of the disease by medical staff and, over a period of time, learns the significant changes it makes to his/her lifestyle and that of significant others.

Goffman argues that this is an isolating experience, and a time when the individual thinks through problems, learns about him/herself and clarifies the situation. It often leads to a new understanding of what is important and worth seeking in life. Obviously, this view is too simplistic to be applied directly to the person with cancer. Whether or not the individual is well enough to consider the important implications of the illness, is dependent on his/her physical condition. It is not always possible for the person with cancer to 'sort out the situation', as the nature of the situation may not be straightforward. The future is often very uncertain and, therefore, future planning is often problematic. However, given time, the person with cancer may learn to adjust to the illness and to reappraise the important aspects of his/her life.

Conclusion — stigma

To conclude, Goffman's work on stigma provides a sound humanistic framework from which to critically analyse the concept of stigma, as applied to the person with cancer. This, in turn, leads to a greater understanding of the complex attitudes of individuals in relation to the nature of stress.

9 Research study design and sample

Research setting and sample

Having completed a theoretical study, an empirical study was carried out in order to create a sound framework for the psychosocial care of persons with cancer.

Methodological triangulation

Several research methods (known as methodological triangulation) were employed, in order to gain an holistic picture of the concept of stress as applied to persons with cancer. It would be naive to presume that a single consistent picture would be obtained by the use of different methods. Indeed, the use of triangulation may uncover variance which would otherwise remain undiscovered by single methods. From a phenomenological perspective, if differences do occur, it is necessary to understand why they are present. This can provide an opportunity to enrich the depth and clarity of explanation of the area under study. Another reason for choosing methodological triangulation for this particular study, was to increase the validity of the results as the problem of researcher bias is avoided. It was essential to take into account the constraints of time and facilities available when selecting the methods for the study, in order to build up as full a picture as possible.

Interviews

In-depth interviews with qualified nursing staff were carried out, making use of an interview guide. This allowed for flexibility of approach in order to gain a deeper understanding of the respondent's perspective. Yet, at the same time, it ensured that all relevant topics were discussed. The interviewer had more freedom to choose when and how to put questions arising naturally from the context of the discussion and how much to explore and probe, whilst still remaining in the framework of topics to be covered. This meant that the interviewer was able to adopt an informal, conversational style with the respondents.

The opening topics of the interview guide were designed to explore the individual's key perceptions regarding cancer, stress and the relationship, if any, between the two concepts. A main feature of the interview guide was an examination of those factors that the individual felt could lead to taxing the ability of persons with cancer to adjust. To create a more detailed picture of the concept of stress as applied to persons with cancer, topics also included factors that may heighten stress, indicators of stress and possible occasions when stress is perceived.

Respondents' perceptions of coping amongst persons with cancer and their patterns of coping were also explored, because of the relationship between stress and coping as proposed by Lazarus (see Chapter 1). The respondents' views regarding the assessment and documentation of stress and coping were discussed. Finally, ways of reducing stress in persons with cancer were examined, in addition to considering the respondents' psychological role.

Non-participant observations

In addition to in-depth interviews, non-participant observation of the nursing admission assessment of persons with cancer was undertaken. Observation serves as a useful qualitative research method, as it allows the researcher to discover what actually occurs, as opposed to the respondent's version of events as related in the research interview. It also enables the researcher to examine implicit or unconscious behaviours that the informant is not always able to describe. Observation allows a study of behaviours that may not be included in the informant's verbal description of a situation. The degree of participation depends on a consideration of what will yield the most meaningful data in the given circumstances.

An observation schedule was developed which included the key psychosocial aspects relating to the nursing care of persons with cancer. The nursing Kardex of the particular health authority concerned was taken into account. The schedule consisted of space to record the person's statements regarding psychosocial aspects and to record patterns of nurses' questioning of persons with respect to these areas. To avoid research bias, it was considered essential to record actual statements where possible, with a precis of relevant verbal information added as soon after completion of the interview as possible. A section was included regarding information given by the nurse, and a distinction was made between physiological and psychosocial areas. The final sheet was designed to provide concise information relating to the patterns of verbal communication (e.g. pattern of questioning and the language used, tone, use of euphemisms for both nurses and persons with cancer). Non-verbal communication of both nurses and persons with cancer was also recorded, due to the importance of this mode of communication. Field notes, which included both methodological notes and analytical notes were made, to provide comparison with the findings and ensure methodological rigour.

Archival sources

Archival sources serve as an important research tool because they are often primary sources, i.e. the material is gathered at first hand. Therefore, they have a direct relationship with people, situations and events that are studied. Hospital records constitute documents that are produced without research in mind. Archival sources can be used in conjunction with other social methods of investigation in order to supplement and validate or cross-check recorded data from one source with data from another. These sources are convenient and time-saving. Archival sources produce descriptive data, as they lend an insight into the perspectives, assumptions, concerns and activities of those who produce them. However, the amount of information is limited to what is available. Thus, the range of material, the quality, the quantity and comparability varies.

For this study, an archival sources schedule was developed from relevant key items from the observation schedule, in addition to key recordable items already present in the nursing Kardex. The research aimed to explore whether the key psychosocial areas pertaining to persons with cancer had been recorded as identifiable needs. If this was the case, the researcher went on to consider whether a plan of action had been recorded and subsequently assessed over time and recorded in the progress notes, together with any preliminary evaluations. Also explored were: whether a record had been made of referrals to other members of the health care team, regarding psychosocial issues and if there were any references to interactions with significant others, in regard to a person's progress. In addition, there was an examination of whether a record had been made of the nature of information given to the person. Finally, it was noted if there were any significant omissions in the nursing Kardex.

Necessary permissions

Permission was gained to carry out a small pilot study on an acute medical ward, specialising in haematology, and to carry out the main study on four general wards of a regional oncology and radiotherapy hospital. Ethical considerations in relation to research were respected and upheld at all stages of the project.

The sample

The sample constituted a non-probability sample. Due to the sensitive nature of the study, individuals with cancer had to be carefully selected, taking into account the views of the consultants and qualified nursing staff. Six consenting persons on the haematology ward (who had been selected by the nursing staff) took part in the pilot study and 30 consenting persons with cancer on the cancer unit (again, selected by the nursing staff) took part in the main study.

Six qualified members of nursing staff on the haematology ward were asked to take part in the pilot study. The remaining four staff, due to their enthusiasm to take part, were subsequently asked. The researcher approached qualified members of nursing staff on the cancer unit and 40 staff were asked to take part in the main study. Staff at both settings varied from enrolled nurses, staff nurses and ward sisters, in order to ensure that a mix of staff were represented and to avoid bias.

The nursing Kardexes of 20 persons with cancer (who had previously consented to observation of their nursing admission assessment) were analysed.

Content analysis — interviews

The main aim was to order, in some way, the elicited common-sense definitions of respondents, in relation to stress and the person with cancer. The categories were not initially grouped or precoded because part of the analysis was precisely whether or not the variables would emerge as patterns reflecting broad themes of common-sense interpretation of the nature of stress in persons with cancer.

Common-sense interpretations are linked to individual nurses' experiences, both past and present, i.e. both professional practice and educational experiences. Although not enough is known about what common-sense knowledge is, or what it means, a framework of common-sense knowledge involves the informal views and the wealth of knowledge that individuals have. This is clearly influenced by experience of interaction with others. Therefore, this research focuses on professional and vocational conceptions of care.

Seven broad category systems were developed (see Tables 9.1, 9.2, 9.3, 9.4, 9.5, 9.6 and 9.7), making use of the constant comparative method (Glaser and Strauss, 1967). These categories were discerned from the subjects' own responses to the areas explored within the interviews. There was no attempt to impose the researcher's own formal taxonomy of categories. The intention in setting up the descriptive categories, was that they should be of value in capturing and representing the important features of respondents' conceptions of the nature of stress in the person with cancer. On the surface, it would appear that all the categories and subcategories developed from individual responses simply reflect the literature. However, on close inquiry, it can be seen that it is not nearly as straightforward and, in fact, there is some fragmentation in perceptions between the theoretical (i.e. theories of stress and related concepts) and common-sense worlds (i.e. the respondents' experiences) shown in the categories and subcategories.

For example, consider the first key category system, causes of stress and category A3. The overall negative view of cancer equalling death was highlighted in the health research literature and also constituted the overriding view perceived by the nurses in relation to stress and persons with cancer. However, the influence of stories about the (cancer) hospital was highlighted and explored by 55% of respondents, but was not evident in the literature. The literature outlined the fear associated with cancer. Yet 50% of respondents were able to discuss the emotion of fear in greater detail and attempted to explore the uncertain world for persons with cancer. In this way, the common-sense interpretation of 50% of respondents make a significant contribution over and above the health research literature.

In category A4, all respondents reflected the literature concerning the general effects of treatment. However, within the subcategory A4.1, not all respondents' views reflected the literature regarding the negative effects of alopecia. In direct contrast to the literature, 25% of respondents argued that the effects of alopecia were minimal compared to issues such as life and death. Thus, the common-sense interpretations of these respondents question the theoretical body of knowledge in relation to the stress associated with alopecia in persons with cancer.

Table 9.1 A categories: causes of stress

category A1	referral to family
category A1.1	effect of cancer upon the relationships between the person with cancer and significant other(s)
category A2	feelings of helplessness/frustration due to dependency
category A2.1	the effects of physical dependency
category A2.2	the effects of psychological dependency
category A3	cancer = death
category A3.1	the influence of stories about cancer
category A3.2	the influence of stories about treatment and the side-effects of treatment
category A3.3	the influence of stories about the hospital itself
category A3.4	the social effects of cancer
category A3.5	the emotion fear, of the unknown/of the uncertain nature of cancer
category A4	treatment and its side effects
category A4.1	the effects of alopecia regarding perceptions of body image
category A4.2	the effects of surgical disfigurement regarding perceptions of body image
category A5	effect of cancer on lifestyle
category A5.1	effect of cancer on job/career
category A5.2	effect of cancer on social life
category A5.3	effect of cancer on future plans
category A6	the effects of pain and fear of addiction to analgesia
category A7	effect of hospitalisation

Table 9.2 B categories: factors that heighten stress

category B1	lack of information
category B1.1	contradictory information
category B2	lack of communication with family/staff
category B3	seeing fellow patients in later stages of illness

Table 9.3 C categories: indicators of stress and coping

category C1	role of experience, having a close helping relationship
category C2	behavioural indicators of stress
category C2.1	physiological indicators of stress
category C3	verbal and non-verbal indicators

Table 9.4 D categories: occasions when stress is likely to be experienced

category D1	key stages in a cancer patient's career
category D1.1	at/soon after diagnosis of cancer
category D1.2	on admission to hospital
category D1.3	during treatment
category D1.4	at time of relapse
category D2	stress as a constant possibility for the cancer patient

Within the B categories of factors that heighten stress, it can be seen that respondents' views regarding lack of information (B1) and lack of communication (B2), reflect the literature relating to the criticism of the support role of the cancer nurse. However, category B3 of seeing fellow patients in the later stages of illness was raised by over 50% of the respondents as heightening stress — yet this factor was not evident in the health research literature. Thus, it can be seen from these examples that, although the categories of subjects' own responses often link directly to the literature, there is also some fragmentation present. This represents, in effect, a distortion of reality between the theory and the common-sense world of results, highlighting differences and similarities between nurses. From a phenomenological perspective, it is much more likely that there does not exist a complementary and totally consistent picture of the stressful world of the person with cancer, between the everyday meanings of the respondents and the theoretical world.

Within the C categories of indicators of stress and coping, 95% of respondents paid attention to behavioural indicators and 55% of respondents to physiological indicators. Within category C1, however, 43% of respondents further develop Lazarus' emphasis on the individual, as they highlighted the importance of getting to know a person over time, in order to assess his/her stress.

Within the D categories of occasions when the person with cancer is likely to experience stress, the respondents' occasions largely

Table 9.5 E categories: perceptions of coping and coping patterns

category E1	coping perceived as postively accepting one's illness
category E1.1	being able to talk openly regarding self
category E1.2	maintaining as near normal a lifestyle as possible
category E2	denial, blocking, 'putting on a front'
category E3	referral to positive approach of 'fighting spirit'
category E3.1	referral to negative approach of 'fighting spirit'
category E4	use of anger and displacement
category E4.1	general inhibition of emotions in hospital
category E5	withdrawal from family and staff
category E5.1	depression
category E6	use of religion
category E6.1	positive effects of religious beliefs
category E6.2	negative effects of religious beliefs
category E7	complementary/alternative therapy
category E8	coping as a changing variable over time and as individualistic
category E9	role of personality regarding coping and effect of cancer upon personality
category E10	use of humour
category E11	positive re-evaluation of self and/or life due to having cancer

reflect those of Weisman (see Chapter 1). Approximately 10% of respondents, however, also raised the issue of stress as a possible constant factor amongst persons with cancer (category D2), which is not considered in the literature.

Within the E categories of the perceptions of coping, the respondents' perceptions with regard to categories E1, E1.1 and E1.2 reflect the 'good copers' identified by Weisman. With respect to the coping patterns, the categories largely reflect the key coping patterns outlined in the literature, such as denial, 'fighting spirit' and withdrawal. However, several categories are not evident within the literature. For example, in subcategory E4.1, 25% of respondents spoke of the negative effect of the hospital environment with regard to the expression of emotions. In category E6.2, approximately 10% of respondents gave specific examples of the negative effects of

Table 9.6 F categories: factors that help to reduce stress including nursing actions

category F1	support from the nurse
category F1.1	the use of counselling skills
category F1.2	the views of nursing staff regarding their support role
category F2	support from family and peers

Table 9.7 G categories: modes of communication regarding stress and factors to help nurses assess stress in the cancer patient

category G1	verbal as key form of communication
category G1.1	advantages and disadvantages of nursing process
category G2	experience as a factor in the assessment of stress
category G3	role of increased training in psychological care, staff support groups
category G4	use guideline questions as systematic means of assessment

religious beliefs. In category E10, regarding the use of humour, this was viewed by 40% of respondents as part of a front (category E2).

Within the F categories of factors that help to reduce stress, including nursing actions, it was found that, in contrast to the health research literature, 88% of the respondents recognised the value of the support role of the nurse, including the use of counselling skills. The constraints present in terms of workload, staffing levels and lack of educational opportunities were discussed by all respondents in relation to their support role (category F1.2). Only 20% of respondents included support from family and peers (category F2), in contrast to the emphasis given in the health research literature. The focus of the respondents was primarily on their support role, hence categories F1, F1.1 and F1.2.

Finally, within the G categories of modes of communication regarding the stress of persons with cancer, 80% of respondents valued verbal means of communication (category G1) as opposed to the use of the nursing process. However, 73% of respondents gave arguments for and against the use of the nursing process (category G1.1). In contrast to the findings of the health research literature, 35% of respondents acknowledged the importance of increased training in psychological care and staff support (category G3), in addition to experience (category G2).

It can be seen that, within these broad category systems, the majority of the responses to the areas explored in the interviews reflect key areas of the literature. However, within a phenomenological perspective, there is not a mirror image reflection, as there are also present significant differences, additions and omissions, from the literature as outlined above. In the everyday world of the person with cancer, it is unlikely that a single picture is perceived by nurses or presented within the literature. Rather, there are likely to exist matches and mismatches of different pictures which attempt to capture a particular experience, which nurses will probably perceive as stressful for the person with cancer.

Themes regarding stress and the person with cancer as perceived by respondents

The themes identified within the interviews (see Table 9.8) represent the clustered views in the categories regarding stress and the person with cancer, as perceived by the nurse respondents. These themes are used only as guidelines to pull together a general outline. In keeping with a qualitative approach, they represent a creative,

Table 9.8 Themes

theme 1	cancer = death (A3)
theme 2	stigma (A3.1–A3.5)
theme3	family (A1–A1.1)
theme 4	feelings of helplessness (A2–A2.2)
theme 5	effect of cancer on lifestyle (A5–A5.3)
theme 6	treatment and its side effects (A4–A4.2)
theme 7	altered body image (A4.1–A4.2)
theme 8	pain (A6)
theme 9	coping and coping patterns (E1–E11)
theme 10	methods of reducing stress (F1–F2)
theme 11	communication patterns regarding stress (G1–G1.1)
theme 12	methods of helping nurses assess stress (G2–G4)

subjective response to the data obtained from the interviews. The major themes are examined in conjunction with the literature, in order to create a firm theoretical framework for the study of stress and the person with cancer, as perceived by cancer nurses.

Theme 1: nurses' views regarding perceptions of cancer

When asked directly about the meaning of stress as applied to the person with cancer, 98% of nurses spoke of cancer being perceived as equal to death for the majority of persons with cancer (cf categories A3–A3.5):

> *People just presume when they've got cancer, that's it... there is really sort of a black picture painted a lot of times.*

One respondent admitted that nurses probably perpetuate this negative picture:

> *Our views are not much better than the general population sometimes.*

This links to the literature regarding attitudes and the tendency of nurses to adopt a general medical approach to cancer. Thus, a mismatch exists, as a medical conception of cancer often overrides a psychological one. Another respondent argued that the negative coverage of the media had subsequent negative effects on people.

When asked if persons with cancer tended to voice negative thoughts directly, most nurses explained that few persons actually express them. However, the respondents spoke of being aware of an individual's underlying concern. Thus, the respondents expressed it more as that which the individuals do not actually say, i.e. an underlying fear. The emotion **fear** and its relationship to the uncertain nature of cancer was raised spontaneously by 50% of respondents when discussing cancer equalling death. Fear was related to the disease itself and fear of the unknown due to the uncertain nature of cancer:

> *Fear of dying, or of pain, of something mutilating happening... afraid of the unknown...*

> *(cf category A3.5)*

The role of intuition here is highly relevant, as it involves a complex phenomenon. Do the nurses genuinely intuit the person with cancer's fears regarding death? Or rather are the respondents' own underlying fears regarding cancer being reflected? Thus, do both create an underlying sensation of acute fear? The respondents are more likely to be making common assumptions regarding cancer, which are largely taken for granted by health care professionals and the public in general. This leads to the adoption of a general negative medical conception of cancer. Hence, the common-sense meanings that nurse respondents attribute to cancer are likely to stem from their personal experiences of everyday life events, and also from the nature of their student education (e.g. not only from the influential role of their nursing experience, but also from anecdotal evidence of neighbours, relatives and friends, as examined by Deeley, 1979). This directly relates to the phenomenological perspective of the importance of the meanings attached to everyday life situations.

Due to the fact that 50% of nurses were able to talk about the emotion of fear, it can be argued that these nurses are adopting a negative stance and, albeit unwittingly, passing these pessimistic views onto the person with cancer (as suggested by Whelan, 1982). How can we promote an optimistic approach in others? The first key step is to have a better understanding of the nature of an individual's attitudes, in order to explore his/her conceptions of cancer.

Theme 2: the concept of stigma

There are direct links between Themes 1 and 2: the negative attitudes associated with cancer, the negative views of the majority of nurses and the fact that, in general, people consider cancer to be stigmatising. The views of most respondents regarding cancer as stigmatising reflects the literature. In particular, 50% of respondents linked the emotion of fear regarding cancer to the taboo surrounding the disease. For example, they explained that few people actually say the word 'cancer'. One respondent commented:

> *Cancer is a taboo subject... people don't like admitting they've got it... It's such a frightening thing... that's it, they're going to die... big mystery.*

> *(cf category A3)*

Pugsley and Pardoe (1988) similarly write of the mystery surrounding cancer, which they argue reveals the intensity and breadth of the emotion fear.

The misconceptions regarding cancer, outlined by most respondents, parallel the myths of cancer presented by Pugsley and Pardoe and Fallowfield (1988). The view of the 'wages of sin' was portrayed by 25% of respondents who revealed the complex emotion of guilt, and the ensuing lowered levels of self-esteem, experienced by women with cancer of the cervix. Also, several respondents recalled elderly persons with cancer who regarded cancer as a shameful, unclean disease and as a result had attempted to keep the fact hidden and not communicate about it to others. The view of 'contagion' was expressed by 33% of respondents, in terms of the social effects of stigma, as they recalled instances of relatives/friends/neighbours of persons with cancer who did not visit, as they feared the disease was infectious.

Several respondents gave specific examples of persons with cancer who had been treated differently by others in social situations. This parallels the work of Goffman (1967) and the way in which the mentally ill are often perceived by others, i.e. as possessing an 'undesired differentness'. For example, these respondents spoke of the distancing effect of people reacting awkwardly in the company of persons with cancer, some to the extreme of actively avoiding them. This reflects the medical model of stereotyping patients into specific categories and attaching labels to them. The medical model emphasises particular traits to the exclusion of the consideration of the patient as a unique individual with his/her own perceptions of the situation.

Fifty-five per cent of respondents developed the concept of stigma further, relating it directly to the hospital itself. Thus, similar to the disease spreading, the negative influence of stigma also spreads to include the care environment of persons with cancer. In effect, it is fear by association, as respondents reported that newly-admitted persons with cancer and relatives voice the fear of the hospital symbolising death. This was due to the direct experience of relatives who had died at the hospital or via the reports of others whose relatives had died there. For example:

> *As soon as you say X hospital, they think cancer... everyone comes out in a box... this is the end of the line now I've come here...*

> *Patients listen to people who say, 'Oh, I know such and such and she never got out of there'... they just know about the cases that don't get better... they don't realise that quite a lot do go home...*

(cf category A3)

Again, several respondents noted that this negative view also extends to health care professionals who express their surprise at how staff at the hospital can work there, 'it must be awful', or, 'they all die there'. This relates to the tendency of staff to adopt a general negative medical conception of cancer.

Forty-two per cent of respondents also spoke of the fear and mystery associated with the treatment itself, and the influence of stories which heighten and grossly distort the side effects of the treatment. This parallels Deeley's (1979) accounts of people exaggerating the effects of cancer itself. For example, the almost universal assumption held by the public was of experiencing nausea, vomiting and alopecia. One respondent explained that a person having radiotherapy to his chest asked when his hair on his scalp would fall out. Another respondent stated how the effects of treatment are exaggerated by other people, and gave an example of a person who came thinking treatment would be awful and found it was not as bad as she had anticipated. A respondent commented that people used not to ride on the top deck of the bus as they passed X hospital, due to fear of 'the rays'.

The fact that all of the respondents considered that there was still a stigma associated with cancer was significant, because it implies that health care professionals have a long way to go before achieving effective health education in cancer. (The prevalent misconceptions regarding cancer, e.g. its automatic association with death, dying and suffering, are still held by a number of nurses.) In effect, health care professionals are adopting a medical conception of cancer. Deeley states that it often takes generations to change people's attitudes regarding the 'scourges of mankind'. If so, which road must we take to ensure that a realistic view of cancer is adopted and fear is minimised? A possible answer lies in the adoption of a humanistic perspective, which centres upon the exploration of a person with cancer's perceptions regarding the nature of his/her illness and treatment (see Chapter 10 for further details).

Once the person has acknowledged that he/she has cancer, an exploration of his/her perceptions regarding cancer is imperative, because the pervading negative views regarding cancer appear to affect all other common causes of concern for the person with cancer. For example, the stigma associated with cancer directly affects the family members and their coping patterns (theme 3) and creates the possibility of difficulties in communication between family members and the person with cancer; feelings of uncertainty link to the compounding effects on the emotion fear and also relate to the sense of a loss of an expected future (theme 5); the stigmatised views of employers regarding cancer and the effects on an individual's job/career; the social effects of having cancer (theme 5); the effects of hospitalisation (theme 9); the common association of pain with cancer (theme 8) and perceived/actual change in body image, i.e. the notion of disfigurement due to treatment (theme 7).

The concept of stigma is likely to form a key area for a person's appraisals of stress and, as a result, also impinges on a diverse range of other themes. As can be seen from this section, this is largely due to the strong negative attitudes surrounding cancer. In particular, all the nurses acknowledged the common association of cancer with death and dying. This has clear links with the general negative medical conception of cancer representing medical failure due to the lack of (to date) an overall medical cure for the disease. Thus, as reflected by the respondents, there often exists, amongst health care professionals in particular, a 'taken for granted' assumption that the person will die from the illness. This often creates a complex fear of the disease, which has a 'compounding effect' and extends to the cancer care environment. It is also affected by other misconceptions, such as those of 'wages of sin' and 'contagion'.

Theme 3: concern for the family

The concept of the family was another key theme discussed fully by respondents and parallel in importance to perceptions of cancer and stigma. Indeed, all respondents spoke of the effects of diagnosis of cancer as having an equally significant effect on every member of the family as for the person with cancer The person with cancer and his/her family were perceived as inherently linked. For example:

...because once they are poorly, that affects everybody else's life, it affects the relationship with your actual partner, also between your children...

The invulnerability of the family member in relation with the rest of the family group is shattered.

(cf categories A1 and A1.1)

The family is a natural choice when asked regarding causes of concern for persons with cancer. Most respondents raised the subject of family immediately after having been asked the general question regarding causes of concern, or after discussing attitudes surrounding cancer. The importance and the centrality of the family are often taken for granted in the literature, as it is commonly assumed that everyone knows the effects upon the family. As a result, the complexity of the effects on the family are often not given sufficient attention and an outline is deemed sufficient. For example, for the purpose of articles, researchers precis the parallel effect on the family, without fully exploring the dynamic and individualistic nature of the concept of the family. In contrast, all respondents were able to expand fully on their perceptions of the effect on the family of persons with cancer and, as a result, revealed some of the intricacies involved. The majority of respondents spoke in almost contrasting terms. They spoke initially in generalised terms of 'the family' as a universal concept and yet were able to subsequently relate specific examples, thus revealing the differences involved.

All respondents emphasised the notion of the person with cancer often voicing concern for the family rather than him/herself. The concept of the family links directly to themes 1 and 2, as all respondents spoke of the person's thoughts regarding the prospect of death, in relation to worrying about his/her significant others. This then led to an exploration of the main perceived worry for 'the children'. Approximately 25% of respondents were able to relate direct examples of mothers, in particular, with young children and the difficulties present. For example, one respondent recalled a woman whose child did not know her, due to prolonged hospitalisation, and cried when she picked him up. The question arises of whether these examples came to light because the respondents were largely all female, were likely to have children themselves and, hence, were able to sympathise with the mothers' predicaments? The other concern commonly raised in connection with children, was the prospect of the person with cancer not being able to see his/her children or grandchildren grow up.

The concerns raised regarding dependents were closely tangible ones. Clearly, this relates to the respondents' common-sense interpretations of the family, which are influenced by their experiences and particular situations. The respondents gave accounts of what was meaningful, for them, in terms of the family and the person with cancer. Thus, their common-sense assumptions regarding worry about the children related specifically to their own fears in the 'what if it were me?' situation (see Chapter 10 for further details).

All respondents, similar to Mishel *et al* (1984) and Stromberg and Wright (1984), were able to outline the contrasting effects on partner relationships with a diagnosis of cancer. An acknowledgement of a 'make or break' situation was voiced. This simplistic picture was further explored by the majority of respondents, who were able to adopt an individualistic approach and gave pertinent examples of how the diagnosis of cancer actually affected particular relationships Several respondents gave a particular example of a police inspector who had recently developed cerebral mestastases, and how he and his family, in particular his wife, were finding acceptance difficult. This was largely due to the significant change in roles and the difficulty in maintaining open communication. In this way, a much greater insight into the pressures was presented.

Theme 4: feelings of helplessness

The theme of helplessness relates directly to theme 3, as the changed roles for the person with cancer have direct implications for that person's significant others. One respondent commented on dependency, 'it upsets the balance of the family'. Sixty-eight per cent of respondents noted, similar to Stromberg and Wright and Welch McCaffrey (1985) that the failure of the person with cancer to carry out normal roles often places increased responsibility on the family. As a result of this, the person with cancer experiences a feeling of dependency and often a sense of failure. A respondent commented:

They feel a burden to their relatives.

They're the strong ones who lead the way... suddenly to have a son or daughter wash their hair...

(cf category A2)

Approximately 25% of respondents also included the likelihood of the expression of the emotion anger and gave specific examples which heightened the depth of the emotions that are possible in everyday situations.

In contrast to the literature, 28% of respondents expanded on the concept of feelings of helplessness by clearly differentiating between physical and psychological forms of dependency. They were able to give specific examples of persons for whom cancer had made significant changes in their ability to care for the daily activities of living, and noted the difficulties present for the persons with cancer, their significant others and also for the nursing staff. In addition, the respondents highlighted the effect on relationships. For example, the effects on partner relationships are parallel to those explored within the theme of the family in the previous section. Similar to Mishel *et al*, approximately one quarter of respondents acknowledged that the key issue regarding psychological dependency for the person with cancer is the perceived loss of control over everyday decisions. The respondents explored this issue primarily in terms of the person's partner taking over the decision-making role.

It can be seen that the respondents' views link directly to a phenomenological approach and Lazarus' transactional model of stress, as the central issue is the role of the human cognition, i.e. **perceived** loss of control, as opposed to a lack of control *per se*. This is in contrast to a response and stimulus approach, which, similar to Seligman's work (1957) on helplessness and experiments with animals, largely fails to take further human variation into account. Mishel *et al*, in contrast to the respondents, focus on the wider issue of the power of the nursing staff in relation to the role of the patient and the ensuing negative effect on the person. Possibly, the nurses did not explore this aspect as they were not consciously aware of their inherent influence over the person's decision-making process and the role of the patient. The question of feelings of helplessness often arose directly from an explanation of the family, hence, an exploration of helplessness in relation to the family was a natural progression.

One respondent gave a clear sociological analysis of her observation of persons with cancer, i.e. that those from the professional classes and women with families/dependents often found physical and/or psychological dependency most difficult, as their change in roles is significant:

> *They can't seem to come down to the level of being ill... they are just completely lost.*

> *(cf category A2)*

Persons from these situations have to change from roles such as maintaining a job with large responsibilities, family responsibilities regarding children and spouse, social and personal responsibilities regarding leisure activities, hobbies and charity work, to the sole role of that of the patient:

> *They have lost all that and see everything is running without them.*

> *(cf category A2.2)*

This links to the literature relating to perceptions of illness and health, in particular, to the view of illness as destructive.

Theme 5: effects of cancer on lifestyle

This theme also directly links to the major theme of the family, as respondents revealed that the family of the person with cancer forms an integral part of his/her life. The concept of loss, which related to the perceived loss of control in the previous theme of helplessness, is discussed in the literature with regard to the loss of an expected future. Fifty per cent of the respondents further developed this concept by relating it directly to the personal loss of plans for the future. The specific examples given by these respondents of persons with cancer whose plans were thwarted, helps to substantiate Northouse's (1981) views regarding the future orientation of today's society, in contrast to the present orientation of survival, required by the person with cancer (see p29).

The examples provided by 25% of respondents gave a sharp reality to the possible effects of cancer on a person's lifestyle. They covered the life span from younger persons who would be unable to form stable relationships; to individuals with young families who would not live to see their children grow up; to those persons of retirement age whose retirement plans would be thwarted. This reflects the respondents' common-sense interpretations, as they are drawing upon effects from their particular situation and experiences that are meaningful, and as a result which represent reality to them. It is interesting to note that only a minority of respondents disagreed and, in contrast, gave specific examples of persons with cancer who had made plans for the future despite their diagnosis and prognosis. These respondents argued that some individuals with cancer planned ahead in order to give themselves something positive to aim for and to 'keep themselves going'. These examples are related more directly to coping patterns.

The effect of cancer on lifestyle was discussed by respondents in relation to the effects on the jobs of persons with cancer. Relating themes of stigma were explored, such as the prevailing negative attitudes of employers and the focus on the financial concerns of the person with cancer and his/her family, which results in increased pressures due to job loss (Stromberg and Wright, 1984; Welch McCaffrey, 1984). Forty-eight percent of the respondents also explored the wider aspects of the effect on the jobs of persons with cancer, by providing specific examples of persons whose jobs were jeopardised or lost, or cases where early retirement or redundancy were enforced. These respondents noted not only financial problems, but also problems adjusting psychologically to a loss of a job, particularly for those persons whose job was a central part of their life. Thus, these respondents provided insight into the emotional effects of cancer, in addition to the practical difficulties of a person's job. Again, this reflects the respondents' common-sense evaluations of the situation.

Theme 6: effects of treatment and side effects

This theme relates directly to the effects of cancer on a person's lifestyle. Several respondents argued that the treatment for cancer often involves prolonged periods of hospitalisation and a period of rest after completion, which has a significant effect on a person's job. This argument is supported by research which found that the stress of persons with cancer, who are receiving radiotherapy, is often associated with the practicalities of having the treatment (Fallowfield, 1988, see p33). The theme of treatment and its side effects also links with the major theme of stigma, as approximately 50% of respondents substantiated the literature, by providing examples of negative connotations associated with the treatment and its side effects (see theme 2 on stigma).

Seventy-five per cent of respondents, similar to the literature with regard to treatment and its side-effects, focused on the negative effects of nausea and vomiting. The same percentage of respondents explored the problems of chemophobia and, in keeping with the research, adopted a stimulus approach (indicative of a medical model) by providing the key stimuli which cause the conditioned response of vomiting in persons with cancer. However, the respondents did not consider the complex role of anxiety and its possible compounding effects on anticipatory nausea and vomiting as presented by Burish and Carey (1986).

As the majority of respondents were able to recall several persons with cancer who experienced chemophobia (and these persons found it extremely difficult to continue with their treatment as a result), this phenomenon is more common than the respondents acknowledged. The literature does not always present a clear picture of the extent of this problem. However, the specific examples given by 50% of the respondents strongly suggest that a significant minority of persons with cancer experience severe problems with their treatment. As one respondent explained:

> *It is difficult, if someone suffers from chemophobia, to have set courses of treatment in hospital, as it affects their lifestyle and is psychologically damaging.*
>
> *(cf category A4)*

Therefore, it is important for the nurse to adopt an humanistic approach, exploring the person's perceptions of treatment on admission to hospital and closely monitoring these perceptions during and after completion of the course of treatment. In this way, more extreme reactions, such as chemophobia, can be spotted and explored fully, in order to help the person learn effective coping patterns and aim to minimise the psychobiological effects of chemotherapy.

The literature reveals the association of the more toxic drugs with a poor quality of life and extreme psychological reactions, e.g. acute anxiety and depression (see p34). Several respondents were able to substantiate this trend as they gave examples of elderly people who felt extremely ill from the effects of treatment, which lead to psychological problems in maintaining the hope of getting better. One respondent argued:

> *They do not see the light at the end of the tunnel.*
>
> *(cf category A4)*

This presents a significant challenge for cancer nurses, in terms of ethical dilemmas regarding treatment and their own important role as patient advocate.

Theme 7: effects of altered body image

This theme connects with the theme of treatment and its side-effects, as all respondents commented on the effects of alopecia on a person's perceptions of body image. In contrast to the literature, 25% of respondents argued that, in their nursing experience, they had not cared for persons with cancer who had suffered from severe problems. The respondents explained that they considered most individuals adjusted to the change over a period of time. Several respondents substantiated their views, by stating that persons with cancer comment that their life is more important than their loss of hair. One respondent noted:

They come to terms with almost anything if it will give them a bit longer and improve their quality of life.

(cf category A4.1)

This argument raises an important point, as surely, the key issue is how the individual appraises alopecia? These respondents failed to adopt an individualistic approach and have not acknowledged, as Salter (1988) states, that whether problems of adjustment will occur depends on the importance placed on hair by the individual (see p69). Instead, they have made the general assumption that most individuals adjust to their hair loss. This reflects the medical model, and the minimisation of the importance of hair loss in comparison to the saving of life. As a result, the respondents are failing to detect possible underlying problems of adjustment in some individuals, and, subsequently, are not meeting their psychological support role.

In contrast to these views, it is encouraging that over half of the respondents acknowledged that, for some individuals with cancer, alopecia was perceived to be stressful, reflecting the literature on alopecia and body image. One respondent commented:

It's a permanent reminder of what's going on.

Several respondents considered it was more difficult for women to adjust to alopecia, due to society's emphasis on beauty and hair. A respondent argued:

It's more psychologically damaging to women, because they are portrayed to be beautiful... if you're bald that's all the community sees — she's wearing a wig... not why is she?... the fact she's fighting for her life...

(cf category A4.1)

Similar to Webb (1985), the respondents outlined society's expectations of appearance with regard to hair. These respondents substantiated their views with specific examples of women that they had nursed. This reflects a phenomenological perspective, due to the emphasis given to an individual's perceptions and experience of alopecia. One respondent commented, similar to Baxley *et al* (1984), that it is often easier for staff to become accustomed to a person's loss of hair than the person him/herself, and gave an example of a man who found the loss of hair follicles on his face upsetting. This emphasises the importance of fully assessing the individual's perceptions with respect to alopecia and body image, together with the importance of empathy in the helping relationship, in order to provide an effective means of support for the person with cancer.

Several respondents highlighted the commonly held assumptions contested by Baxley *et al* (1988), as they explained that alopecia does not often present a problem for men. However, one respondent adopted a humanistic approach and acknowledged that perhaps for some men, their problems remained underlying ones, due to society's expectations regarding masculine roles. These findings have important nursing implications, as it is probable that a significant proportion of men with cancer are not receiving the same amount of attention that their female counterparts are given with regard to adjustment to altered body image. This reiterates the value of a humanistic approach in which the nurse and the person with cancer — male or female — explore the person's perceptions of changed body image.

Within the theme of altered body image, the effects of surgical disfigurement were outlined by 50% of the respondents, particularly in relation to persons with mastectomy. These respondents linked this theme to the theme of the family, as they focused on the effects of a changed body image with regard to partner relationships. They gave specific examples of the negative effects of a mastectomy on the individual and on relationships between the individual and partner. By relating the theme to particular individuals and their experiences, these respondents developed a more phenomenological approach, in contrast to a restrictive medical oriented problem approach.

A significant omission by the majority of respondents was an exploration of the effects of an altered body image on sexual relationships and sexuality. This subject was only briefly mentioned in the literature in relation to persons with loss of a limb. However, in contrast to the literature, several of the respondents adopted a phenomenological approach and, thus, were able to give specific examples of persons who experienced stress, due to their perceived inability to form sexual relationships with a partner. Several respondents, reflecting the literature, mentioned that, in general, for persons with a colostomy, maintaining intimate relationships was difficult. Respondents were not asked directly about the effects of altered body image on sexual relationships and sexuality. Nevertheless, the fact that none of the respondents raised the subject of sexuality at all, and that very few respondents explored the effects of altered body image on sexuality, poses significant nursing implications. If the literature in this area is taken into consideration, then the inherent links between an altered body image and sexuality become apparent.

Could it be that respondents, similar to nurses in general as argued in the literature, tend not to discuss this subject with persons experiencing an altered body image, because of negative attitudes and a lack of psychological knowledge? In keeping with a medical approach, unless a person with cancer experiences severe problems and is able to vocalise these, it is highly likely that the subject is not raised and, as a result, a person's support needs are not adequately met.

Theme 8: pain and analgesia

The theme of pain has direct links with the major theme of stigma, as several respondents noted the common association of cancer with pain. Pain is often experienced and anticipated by persons with cancer. Several respondents also explained that persons with cancer voice their concern particularly with regard to the prospect of dying in pain. This reflects the work of McCaffrey (1983) (see p57). All respondents discussed pain as a major cause of stress. One respondent gave a significant contrast between pain in childbirth and cancer pain. In the former, there is usually a positive result, whereas in the latter, all the person has is a constant reminder that he/she has something which could lead to death. Several respondents acknowledged that pain also causes stress for the individual's family, which is in keeping with the research findings on chronic cancer pain (see p58).

Twenty-five per cent of respondents acknowledged the psychological element involved regarding pain, as they argued that pain is heightened in the presence of anxiety. They gave several examples of specific individuals with cancer to substantiate their argument. The views of these respondents reflect a phenomenological perspective, as they emphasised the individual and his/her perceptions regarding pain. They acknowledged the highly qualitative and individualistic nature of pain, as highlighted in the literature .

A quarter of the respondents also gave specific examples of persons with cancer, for whom it was difficult to achieve pain control, and the influence of fear and anxiety in accentuating their pain. 'Pain becomes the focal point of their lives' (cf category A6). This highlights the findings of Bonica (1984) regarding persons with recurrent cancer (see p57). One respondent commented:

Sometimes patients come in on fantastic doses of analgesia, then something can happen and they have a good cry and the pain might be better.

(cf category A6)

The respondents also explained that persons often become preoccupied with their pain and lose interest in social activities to an extent that their experience of pain dominates their lives.

Although these respondents adopted a phenomenological approach, as they acknowledged the individualistic and qualitative nature of pain, none of the respondents explored the wider cultural influences on perceptions of pain, as highlighted in the literature. This is probably due to the fact that there were not any direct questions asked regarding cultural factors. Also, all persons with cancer in the research setting came from a similar geographical area, hence, cultural factors were not likely to be a central aspect regarding perceptions of pain in this study.

It is encouraging that 25% of the respondents directly contrasted the findings of Bonica (1984), with respect to the general lack of concern amongst health care professionals regarding pain. These respondents were able to give specific examples of pain and persons with cancer, thus revealing an empathic approach. These respondents took into account the individual and his/her perceptions of pain, acknowledging the individual as the expert regarding the meanings attributed to his/her experience of pain. This is in contrast to the medical model, which assumes the superior role of the professional as expert in assessing the person with cancer's pain and prescribing analgesia accordingly.

Several respondents, in contrast to the literature, also raised the subject of the problems associated with persons with cancer fearing the possibility of becoming addicted to their analgesia. These respondents outlined the negative influence of the media, and occasionally the medical staff, with regard to opiates. One respondent stated:

Some patients are frightened of taking analgesia so they live with the pain uncomplainingly.

(cf category A6)

The fear of addiction to analgesia was not explored at all in the literature reviewed. However, fear of addiction to opiates represents a significant factor and is likely to become increasingly so, with the care of persons with auto immune deficiency syndrome.

Factors that heighten stress

Table 9.9 Factors that heighten stress

if a person feels isolated
*if a person cannot talk to his/her family
*if an individual's family withholds information from him/her
*if an individual does not receive information regarding the course of action whilst he/she is in hospital
*if a person receives contradictory information regarding his/her progress and course of treatment
if staff are not experienced enough
personality clashes with fellow patients
if a person does not get on with other people around him/her
*seeing fellow patients in later stages of illness
*being in the same room as someone who is very ill and then when the person is subsequently moved out of the room
if a person is transferred to another ward
if a doctor does not return to see an individual as promised
if treatment is not given on time
if there is no welcome for a person on admission and he/she has to wait a long period of time for a bed
if an individual is not having any active treatment and is awaiting the doctor's decision regarding subsequent treatment
if a person is unable to have the food he/she wants and if a meal is poorly served
if aspects of an individual's care are not carried out how he/she would like
if a person has to stay in hospital longer than anticipated
changing nurses when a person has begun to know a particular member of staff
if treatment/medication has changed

* Voiced by more than 50% of respondents

All respondents outlined a diverse range of factors which they perceived heightened a person with cancer's stress. This clearly reflects a phenomenological perspective, due to the individualistic approach adopted. Respondents were most likely to give emphasis to those factors which reflected their particular experiences. Table 9.9 is a table of factors involved.

The factors marked with an asterisk are those that were voiced by more than 50% of the respondents. It can be seen that problems relating to communication were regarded as key factors which heighten stress for the person with cancer.

Factors regarding occasions when stress is experienced

All respondents were able to give a variety of occasions when the person with cancer is likely to experience stress. Similar to Table 9.9, individual differences are present, which are based on the respondents' everyday experiences. Table 9.10 illustrates the factors involved.

Table 9.10 Factors regarding occasions when stress is experienced

prior to diagnosis when the cause of the problem is unknown (waiting for results of investigations)
*at the time of diagnosis
*on first admission to hospital and on readmission
at the start of treatment
*whilst the person is having treatment
awaiting the response of treatment
*on discharge from hospital
*at the time of recurrence
at visiting time, visitors asking questions and the person having to be optimistic in front of the visitors
during doctors' rounds
*at night-time (due to the fact that there is more time to think for a person to think about him/herself and his/her situation than in the day-time when there is much more activity)
*immediately prior to an outpatient appointment

* Voiced by more than 50% of respondents

Again, the factors marked with an asterisk are those that were voiced by more than 50% of the respondents. However, several respondents explained that they perceived having cancer as being potentially stressful for all or most of the time:

If it was me I would be worrying every verse end... any reminder of their situation or vulnerability.

The whole way along even when they're in remission I wonder if any ever get to the point where they are no longer stressed.

I can't pinpoint when there is any time when you can't say with cancer patients, that there isn't a stressful time... I'm not saying all patients are laid in a state of stress, constantly 24 hours... but each and every day can be stressful.

(cf category D2)

Key indicators of stress

Forty-three per cent of respondents emphasised that they considered it important to know the person with cancer, in order to assess whether they are experiencing stress. This reflects an emphasis on the individual as the expert with respect to him/herself and his/her particular situation. Sixty-three per cent of respondents gave value to verbal means of communication regarding stress, i.e. whether a person with cancer is able to confide his/her worries:

Just by experience you learn to know by talking to the patient and with the knowledge that people react to stress in different ways...

(cf category C1)

Several respondents also noted that stress can be indicated if persons with cancer ask a lot of questions and are repetitive; or talk for a long time but do not say very much and it is difficult to end a conversation; or hide what they are saying in another sentence; or give 'yes' and 'no' answers. In addition, approximately 25% of respondents spoke of much more subtle indicators which are almost intuitive:

You just know.

You get an impression.

It's an insight.

(cf category C1)

Ninety-five per cent of respondents gave explanations which often included behavioural factors and, in particular, included a change in behaviour:

- 'going over the top', i.e. extremely high in spirits;
- **or** respondents spoke of persons with cancer who are extremely quiet and often do not respond to questions or mix with other people;
- **or** respondents spoke of individuals with cancer who may be unusually chatty or complain about lots of things or something non-specific.

The importance of non-verbal cues was noted by thirty-two per cent of respondents. These focused on the use of body language, such as crying, wringing hands, looking sad, door closed when usually open, holding your attention longer than is needed, looking very worried or fidgeting. One respondent commented:

You just have to look at them to know...

(cf category C3)

Fifty-five per cent of respondents emphasised the physiological indicators of stress, such as 'not eating' and 'not sleeping', in keeping with a response-based approach to stress. Approximately 25% of respondents explained that, at night, persons who are experiencing stress are often unable to sleep. They may get up and ask for a cup of tea and/or smoke a cigarette, or shut themselves off in the day room. One respondent explained that, at night, persons symptoms are heightened, hence, they feel worse. Another respondent noted that they give a 'rejection face' i.e. 'come and see me' is written in their faces. Physiological indicators noted by these respondents were not valued in isolation, but were taken into account with other forms of assessment of stress, i.e. non-verbal cues, verbal communication.

Several respondents argued that pain is an indicator of stress. One respondent explained that it is difficult to ascertain whether pain causes stress or vice versa (see Chapter 6). Several respondents were careful to point out that indicators of stress are individualistic and vary from person to person:

They vary from person to person and it also depends on the time the person catches them and vice versa.

(cf category C1)

Theme 9: coping

Perceptions and indicators of coping

Fifty-five per cent of the respondents equated coping with cancer as being able to manage the illness on an everyday basis. This also closely involved the notion of persons accepting their illness; adopting a positive outlook; placing an emphasis on action as opposed to passivity and feeling in control over their situation. It can be seen that this reflects a behavioural approach (indicative of a biomedical model and the work of Weisman on coping, 1979; see p14), in terms of 'good copers' who are optimistic, confront reality and take appropriate action. For example:

> *To live their life and not let cancer rule it.*

> *They appreciate that they are not well and accept their limitations, but they do as much as they can...*

> *...making the best of it... feeling that you are still to some extent in control of your life and that it's still worth living...*

> *(cf category E1)*

A key factor raised by 68% of respondents, was the ability of persons with cancer to talk openly to significant others and/or staff regarding their emotions and concerns. Thus, the nurses' overall views regarding coping convey a judgmental approach, which contrasts directly to the individualistic approach of Lazarus (i.e. coping involves efforts to manage stressful demands regardless of outcome, see p15).

The findings raise ethical implications, as it is likely that nurses who adopt (albeit subconsciously in some cases) a similar view of coping to that of Weisman (1979), may adopt a negative stance towards persons with cancer who cope in different ways from 'good copers'. It is possible that such persons may be treated in perhaps more subtle ways as a 'difficult patient', as presented by Stockwell (1972) (see p15). For example, 'good copers' tend to be seen as those who adopt a 'fighting spirit', are cheerful, optimistic regarding their outlook and remain active, thus being more amenable to nursing staff. In contrast, 'poor copers' are likely to be seen as those who withdraw into themselves and become non-communicative, or become depressed and communicate emotions such as anger and frustration to nursing staff. Over a given period of time, they will probably be viewed in a negative light and constitute a nursing 'problem'. Indeed, those persons who, in Weisman's terms, are 'poor copers' may not receive the support they require in order to help them adjust to their illness.

Equally, it can be argued that the behaviourist notions of good and bad also carry the implication of achievers and non-achievers, superiors and inferiors, which fails to respect the individual and his/her way of managing illness (i.e. the notion that there exists a standard acceptable form of coping which involves being cheerful and optimistic, to which we are expected to comply). In contrast, a phenomenological approach, reflected by Lazarus (1984), focuses on the individual and explores coping patterns, without adopting a judgmental approach, in order to gain an understanding of the reasons behind the individual's way of coping. The nurses' general views regarding coping detract from an individualistic approach encouraged by Lazarus and lead to a stereotyping of individuals with cancer. As a result, the uniqueness and complexity of an individual's personality and patterns of coping are not fully appreciated.

Key indicators of coping and non-coping in the person with cancer

The majority of respondents acknowledged that it is difficult to assess whether a person with cancer is coping in hospital, especially when being admitted:

> *You can judge how they appear to be getting through a normal day... but you can't ever fully know how accurate you'd be.*

(cf category C2)

Several respondents explained that they asked persons directly how they were coping:

> *...patients can come out with all this . [talk about how they have sorted it out and feel settled in their mind] yet underneath they are not at all... some people are good actors.*

(cf category C2.2)

Forty-three percent of respondents explained that it was essential to get to know the person well, over a period of time, in order to assess coping or non-coping. They acknowledged the centrality of the individual. Several respondents also emphasised the central role of relatives, as they appreciated that the relative often knows the person well, and can detect his/her patterns of coping or non-coping.

This section links to the section on indicators of stress, due to the similarity of the key categories. Likewise, the role of intuition was explained by several respondents who stated that it is:

Just a feeling.

You just know... it's difficult to put into words.

(cf category C1)

There exists a contrast between the overall views and the more specific views related to direct nursing experience when considering the concept of coping and persons with cancer. The two conflicting models reflect the focus of the approach as a macro approach, presented by the stimulus and response-based models of stress, and the behavioural approach of the nurses' overall views regarding coping. However, if a more in-depth micro approach is taken, the individualistic approach adopted by 43% of the nurses reflects Lazarus' transactional model of stress in relation to coping. It is important to note the complexity of the concept of coping, and the probability of respondents having 'black and white' views. Instead, it is probably more in keeping with a phenomenological perspective for the nurses to have conflicting views, and it is essential to fully explore the mismatching of these perceptions, in order to contribute to a greater understanding of coping and persons with cancer, as perceived by cancer nurses.

Introduction to coping patterns

Seventy per cent of respondents stated that individuals with cancer cope in different ways. The majority of respondents also gave a diverse range of coping patterns and were able to give specific examples of persons whom they had nursed. The fact that coping changes over time as a person's health status varies, was also noted by 70% of respondents:

Yes. I think it changes according to how well they feel themselves... a bad day... something has gone wrong, then perhaps they may not cope as well.

If treatment is going well they are usually quite high and hopeful — if they are ill and things aren't going right, then they are going to be down.

(cf category E8)

The different coping patterns put forward by the nurses do not represent direct forms of coping. Instead, they reflect more indirect, cognitive forms of coping, in keeping with key factors regarding cognitive forms of coping. These cognitive patterns of coping, when analysed with Lazarus' key factors (see p10), reveal the appropriateness of more indirect forms of coping. For example, when faced with the ambiguous nature of cancer and the powerful and stigmatising general beliefs about cancer, direct forms of coping, such as attack, are not possible.

Denial

Denial was considered by 78% of respondents as a more common form of coping for persons with cancer in the early stages of their illness. Several respondents reflected Lazarus' view (1984) that denial is useful when it is not possible to do anything constructive. The respondents argued that it is not realistically possible for persons with cancer to think about their illness all the time, as they need a period of respite. However, several respondents recalled a minority of individuals who continued to deny their illness. These respondents, similar to Weisman (1979), argued that in the terminal stages of illness, denial is inappropriate, unrealistic and harmful, in terms of being emotionally exhausting. Thus, a judgmental approach was adopted by a minority of nurses with regard to the long-term use of denial.

One respondent explained that the person knows what is the matter, but does not want to be told that it is cancer. Another respondent argued that individuals who deny their illness refuse to let the disease have any influence on their lives. Several respondents spoke of persons with cancer who use euphemisms for the word 'cancer'. One respondent noted that a person could cope with a wart in the bladder, but it was much more difficult to cope with the fact that he/she has cancer. 'Wart' is easier to say and is not stigmatised. Another respondent expressed denial in terms of individuals not mentioning that they have cancer at all, or not talking about their illness. Several respondents stated that some individuals with cancer may keep questioning different members of staff, to see if anyone will give them a different answer.

The following examples of denial relate to the nurses' personal experiences of particular individuals with cancer:

A man who was an entertainer and had many showbiz friends denied his illness by talking about his next contract and recording.

A health visitor who carried on working despite severe dyspnoea and frequent hospitalisation for pleural aspirations.

A lady wouldn't accept that she had bone metastasis and verbalised it as arthritis.

(cf category E2)

Approximately 25% of respondents were careful to explain the differences between denial and 'putting on a front', which stems from their everyday experiences and involves 'seeing through' the image of the person with cancer. They explained that if a person is denying, that individual tends not to talk about the illness at all. However, if a person is putting on a front, the individual is able to talk about the illness but often maintains that he/she is all right. Several respondents spoke of individuals 'putting on a mask', in an attempt to hide their true feelings:

> *They put on a brave face on the surface, but underneath they are just a wreck really.*

> *It is for everybody else, especially the nurses and they can be acting the whole time except when they are on their own.*

> *(cf category E2)*

One respondent related putting on a front to men with cancer who appear:

> *...to put on a 'tough face' and they tend to hide behind it, especially when visitors come... they put up a barrier and it is difficult to get beneath.*

> *(cf category E2)*

Use of strong emotions

Sixty-three per cent of respondents related the use of strong emotions to the use of anger. Although these respondents had had experience of individuals who coped by the use of anger, 28% of respondents argued that, for the majority of these persons, this was not the case. These respondents spoke of the restricting environment of hospitals which makes it difficult to vent anger:

> *Patients are bound to have thousands of emotions bubbling under the surface, but society expects you to present a face...*

> *(cf category E4.1)*

Several respondents explained that persons with cancer react differently, when in hospital, to when they are within their home environment:

> *We only see the 'topside' of people... they may give us a distorted view of the emotions they display within a hospital setting.*

> *They bottle it up... they do not want to break down in front of nurses and relatives.*

> *(cf category E4.1)*

This relates to the internalised social values regarding the expected behaviour of the person with cancer as a patient. One respondent pointed out that strong emotions are something people are often ashamed and embarrassed about, and if they do occasionally display these emotions, they tend to apologise. The general inhibitions of emotions by persons with cancer has links with the coping patterns of 'putting on a front'.

Nearly 50% of respondents were able to give specific examples of people they had nursed who had expressed their anger in the form of displacement on to the staff or family. For example:

> *One man became increasingly angry with his wife as his discharge date grew nearer.*

> *A chap, one of those people labelled cancer phobic, has now been confirmed as having cancer of the pancreas.. is very aggressive towards the staff...*

> *(cf category E4)*

Several respondents explained that some individuals with cancer may feel bitter with their general practitioners for not diagnosing their illness promptly. Another respondent argued that sometimes anger may be displaced on to fellow patients:

> *You get a lot of patients who are... on the defence all the time and if they are in a bay with somebody who's sort of perhaps demented or 'not all there', then they take it out on that patient instead of taking it out on themselves.*

> *(cf category E4)*

One respondent commented:

> *...sometimes it helps if people can blame it on someone... it makes it easier to deal with...*

> *(cf category E4)*

Withdrawal and depression

Thirty-three per cent of respondents were able to give examples of persons with cancer who became withdrawn and 38% of respondents explained that some individuals subsequently became depressed. The examples frequently included persons who withdrew into themselves and did not communicate with family or staff:

> *One patient, when he was told his diagnosis lay on his bed and did not communicate at all with the staff.*

> *(cf category E5)*

One respondent commented that, sometimes, due to treatment taking place over a long period of time and adverse reactions, individuals with cancer find the situation difficult. For example, if they cannot eat, then they become withdrawn. Another respondent similarly noted that withdrawal is common when a person feels that he/she is not improving and has been in hospital for a long period of time. One respondent stated, however, that she considered it was uncommon for such individuals to cut themselves off completely, as, to some extent, they often view the staff as their only hope. It can be seen that approximately 38% of respondents' examples were drawn directly from their everyday experiences of persons with cancer, reflecting a phenomenological approach.

'Fighting spirit'

The use of a 'fighting spirit' of persons with cancer was reported by 70% of respondents, who were able to give specific examples of individuals who had adopted this pattern. The majority of these respondents viewed it as a positive means of coping. The evidence presented by Greer, Morris and Pattingale (1979) regarding longer survival rates for those persons with cancer who adopt a 'fighting spirit' (see p21), was reinforced by several respondents, as they recalled individuals who had lived longer than staff had anticipated. These persons with cancer had been determined to carry on living and had not resigned themselves to their illness. One respondent linked a positive attitude and doing things to help themselves to the use of complementary therapy (see p119). Another respondent noted that people have returned to hospital after having had treatment with money they have raised for the hospital, as a means of expressing their thanks to the staff for helping them.

Twenty-five per cent of respondents explained this coping pattern in terms of the person with cancer being determined to beat the illness and to not let it take him/her over:

> *...patients verbalise that cancer isn't going to rule their lives. I'm going to get the better of this, it isn't going to beat me...*

> *(cf category E3)*

One respondent recalled individuals who kept returning to hospital, each time in advancing stages of deterioration, but who were determined to carry on. Several respondents spoke of a 'fighting spirit' in terms of ways in which a person with cancer can regain the control over those areas of his/her life that were lost on diagnosis of cancer, i.e. a means of becoming less vulnerable:

> *...if you decide you're going to fight, then you're trying to bring it back within your control.*

> *(cf category E3)*

This links to the concept of helplessness (see Chapter 7) and the central role of an individual's perceptions.

Several respondents noted that younger persons with cancer tend to adopt this pattern, as they have not lived their lives to the full and are often determined to overcome it:

> *One young lad who is very positive and continues to play sport.*

> *One young man who was self-employed worked right through his treatment.*

> *(cf category E3)*

A respondent commented that someone with a 'fighting spirit' can also jolly everybody else along, i.e. a person's positive approach rubs off on to other people. Twenty per cent of respondents also explained that support from fellow patients and family helped individuals adopt a more positive approach towards their illness:

> *They often get support from other members of the family... you get people who decide they are going to fight it and become very aggressive towards their disease, and it's not going to beat me...*

> *(cf category F2)*

The respondents highlight the positive effect of 'counter-harm resources', outlined by Lazarus (see p5), which help to reduce stress and also help to determine the nature of the coping action.

Religious beliefs and the use of prayer

A judgmental approach was adopted by sixty-three per cent of respondents, who clearly stated the positive effects of religious beliefs amongst persons with cancer. Several respondents gave examples of persons with cancer who found their religion helped them through their illness and treatment:

> *There was a Catholic lady and she sort of found it comforting... she also found it a lot better to talk to the bloke... she used to speak to him and also people from the congregation came to see her.*

...prayer is very comforting for some patients... one lady used to read her prayer book and a group of patients used to sit together and read prayers.

One patient had a faith healer and it encouraged the patient to get on with his treatment... the fact that somebody had come in and shown he'd got faith in them he managed to get up and be more active.

(cf category E6.1)

These respondents highlighted a form of cognitive manoeuvres presented by Morris, Buckley and Blake (see p21).

However, in contrast to the general positive stance taken by respondents, a significant minority argued that for persons with religious beliefs, it can have a negative effect. One respondent explained that it depends at what stage in life a person believes.

The same respondent gave an example of a person with cancer who was deeply religious and felt that God was not listening to her calls for a miracle, which greatly added to her stress.

If you believe its God's will then you can often accept it peaceful. It's when you feel that it's not right and you have been a good Christian all your life and now God's not answering... it can be very destructive.

(cf category E6.2)

Another respondent recalled a nun who lost her faith, as she felt abandoned by God.

It can be seen that religious beliefs parallel Lazarus' recognition of the importance of an individual's general belief patterns, as these beliefs did not only influence the person's appraisals of stress, but also influenced coping pattern(s).

Complementary/alternative therapy

Thirty-eight per cent of respondents explained that the use of other therapies was uncommon. These respondents were able to give several examples of persons with cancer who were in the minority and used forms of complementary therapy. Their use was seen to have a positive benefit in terms of helping the individual to cope by gaining control over the illness, as opposed to feeling helpless (similar to the positive effects of using a 'fighting spirit'):

They are hoping to give themselves some extra elastic to handle these things...

...for some patients it opens the door to other things... it puts the onus on them — to lead a more healthy life and to try to take steps to have a better diet...

One patient, his GP had taught him to self hypnotise himself to control his breathing and thus relax himself whilst receiving chemotherapy.

(cf category C7)

This reflects the importance of the individual and the recognition of the active role possible in the illness, as opposed to the passive patient role representative of a medical approach.

Approximately 25% of respondents spoke of individuals with cancer who made use of the Bristol diet and found it helped them:

One or two ladies... they'll be on the Bristol diet as well as having radiotherapy, high dose vitamins and things like that... mentally it helps them that's all it does, helps them through the treatment.

One respondent commented that for one person it was a:

...lifeline... something to cling to...

(cf category C7)

Several respondents mentioned relaxation classes that were being held at the hospital. However, one respondent stated that few people were interested and the men reacted negatively. They were:

...totally against it as they considered it to be a sort of wet thing to do.

(cf category C7)

One respondent argued that often relatives are more interested in homoeopathy than the person with cancer. She gave an example of a man who had mistletoe injections in his tumour site for his daughter, as she believed it to be helpful. Another respondent noted that few individuals with cancer in the north of England use complementary or alternative therapy for a variety of reasons: education, availability, resources, interest and motivation. In contrast, the respondent argued that in the south, particularly in London, persons with cancer are encouraged to do positive things to help themselves. Another respondent similarly stated that it depends on education and geographical location, as the Bristol diet is on the hospital menu in London. She noted that most individuals tread the middle line and 'dabble' with complementary medicine.

These respondents clearly adopted a behavioural approach due to the stereotyping of persons with cancer, in contrast to a phenomenological perspective with the emphasis on the individual. Twenty-five per cent of respondents acknowledged that few opt out totally from traditional medical care, as they trust the doctor. This reflects the power of orthodox medicine within our westernised society. Several respondents gave an example of a person with cancer who had been an exception to the rule. For example:

> *There was a young man... who was diagnosed as a teratoma and he decided to opt out... he went down to Bristol... it didn't work and he got quite a massive recurrence and sort of like ate humble pie... came back and had chemotherapy like he would have had...*

(cf category E7)

Several respondents argued that the reason for the lack of use of complementary therapies is not always due to the individual, but to the staff's lack of pursuit and encouragement of different therapies. One respondent gave an example of relaxation tapes which she had sorted out, but were not readily accessible to persons with cancer, so were not widely used and encouraged. She argued:

> *We're too eager to reach for the tablets, not meditation or perhaps a different drink at night.*

(cf category E7)

Another respondent similarly noted:

> *We don't encourage enough distraction... we have to do more...*

(cf category E7)

These respondents highlighted the criticisms presented in the literature (see p37) of the current lack of psychological support given by cancer nurses.

Positive aspects of having cancer

Forty per cent of respondents replied affirmatively that, for some persons with cancer, there are positive aspects of having cancer. These were often voiced in the form of being optimistic and making plans for the future, by doing things with family and close friends; in effect, a re-evaluation of their lives.

One respondent explained that it highlights that which you have nearly lost (i.e. your life) and some individuals with cancer go out and do more things than they would have done previously:

If they have been working, sleeping, not perhaps really living... they get a bit of a jolt to take things a bit easier... just take time out... I'm going to change for the better...

There's probably s lot of positive things happening, for example, a marriage brought closer together, but it's difficult to identify when you have got everything else on your plate.

...they see things that you'd never notice... I think trivial things no longer exist and you do have a different outlook on life...

(cf category E11)

The latter respondent recalled an incident when she had complained to a person with cancer about the cold morning, and the individual replied that to him it was a beautiful morning because he had survived the night. Another respondent noted that persons with cancer often learn a lot about themselves and their strengths, i.e. they have been through the stress of diagnosis of cancer and are now coming out the other side. The respondent regarded this as being positive, as they know exactly how they have got where they are.

These respondents reflect Lazarus' individualistic approach, as they similarly acknowledge that appraisals of stress need not necessarily be construed as solely harmful, but may also be seen as beneficial. This clearly depends on the individual and his/her particular situation.

Use of humour

The fact that humour is often used as a front to hide real emotions was explained by 40% of respondents:

People make funny things out of situations... the temptation is to ignore the underlying currents, yet on the other hand be careful not to read too much into things.

(cf category E10)

Several respondents commented that sometimes, when an individual is the 'life and soul' and always bright, it is difficult to know whether the person is being his/her normal self or putting on a 'big act':

Some patients put on a brave face and try and keep everyone else going well.

...you tend to think they're coping well and underneath they are perhaps finding it difficult to cope...

Ladies with a mastectomy sometimes say, 'Oh look at me I'm all lopsided... I'll be falling to one side'... this is covering up, 'Oh crumbs look at this, it's awful...

(cf category E10)

Several respondents recalled persons with cancer who had a good sense of humour and liked to joke and make people smile. One respondent explained that if people can get together and have a laugh and a joke, they can use it as a way of encouraging everybody to get along well together, i.e. a form of support. However, another respondent argued that humour sounds 'particularly sick' if it has gone 'over the top', as it 'falls flat and sounds unnatural.' She added, 'you expect people to be down if you tell them they have cancer' (cf category E10). This view reflects a behavioural approach, as it conveys the stereotyping of persons with cancer and also implies the expectation that their behaviour is a static concept.

Role of personality and coping

Forty-eight per cent of respondents acknowledged that personality is a complex concept and it is difficult to assess whether coping reflects personality, or whether diagnosis of cancer changes a person's personality. Several respondents agreed that this is difficult to assess if the nurse does not know what the person is normally like (i.e. prior to the onset of cancer). Approximately 25% of respondents argued that persons with cancer may change personality due to their illness. Some individuals may react 'out of character'. One respondent recalled several persons with cancer who 'tended to give up' but who previously had 'very strong personalities'. Another respondent explained:

The bright bubbly person who has faced knocks and started life again, does not necessarily mean he will be able to face having cancer.

(cf category E9)

In contrast:

The introvert who you might worry about suicide threats may cope admirably...

She concludes:

It's difficult... I don't think you ever truly know a patient...

Another respondent noted:

...you get your surprises as well and that is even sadder because if they are normally copers, they feel doubly inadequate if they can't cope with their own illness.

(cf category E9)

These respondents recognised the changing nature of a person's personality, in accordance with their experiences in everyday life.

However, several respondents argued that personality is a more static concept:

There'll always be non-copers, no matter whether it's a leaking radiator or an amputated leg... some types just can't cope.

If someone is an organised, sensible person then they are likely to take things in their stride... [but] if they normally go to pieces if the bus is late... they are not going to react as well as the other person.

(cf category E9)

In contrast to the other respondents, these respondents, who represented a significant minority, adopted a behavioural approach by stereotyping individuals and implying their passive, unchanging nature.

Themes 10 and 12: psychological support role of the cancer nurse

It is encouraging that all respondents spontaneously raised the importance of the support role of the cancer nurse as a means of reducing stress in a person with cancer (theme 10). For example:

To be their advocate... also their mother hen...

To become a friend.

To act as go-between amongst different members of the health care team.

To act as a lifeline for the patient.

(cf category F1.2)

Sixty-eight per cent of respondents, in keeping with the literature (see p43), spoke of the use of communication and counselling skills and the giving of appropriate information:

To put them in touch with other people with the same illness.

(cf category F1)

> *To recognise everyone is an individual in how they want to be supported and if they gain support from talking to the cleaner, that's fine.*
>
> *(cf category F1.2)*
>
> *To be consistent in care... all carers need to talk on the same wavelength.*
>
> *(cf category F1)*

All the respondents acknowledged the importance of their support role, even if they were not able to carry it out fully in practice, due to a number of constraints. In this way, these nurses are a significant step further forward from the nurses presented in earlier research findings (see p41). Sixty-eight per cent commented on the positive side-effects of talking with, and listening to, persons with cancer, in terms of reducing the persons' stress. However, only 33% of respondents highlighted the literature findings and acknowledged (albeit implicitly via the need for more training) that cancer nurses, as a whole, have a significant way to go before they are recognised by persons with cancer as core support givers.

Only 20% of respondents reflected previous research findings (see p40) by commenting on the value of the family as a key source of support for the person with cancer. For example:

> *To appreciate that people open up to relatives rather than to a nursing uniform.*
>
> *Bringing the relatives in with the care if they want to.*
>
> *Allowing members of the family to spend longer periods of time with the patient.*
>
> *(cf category F2)*

All respondents openly spoke of the constraints on them, which made the actual implementation of their support role extremely difficult in everyday clinical practice:

> *The support role could be improved as you've not always got the time that you would like to have.*
>
> *Psychological support is often missed a bit due to workload.*
>
> *(cf category F1.2)*

Several respondents explained that they felt governed by rule and regulations, which made it difficult to be the patient's advocate at times. One respondent spoke of the role of personal mood and subsequent guilt feelings about job performance when off duty. Approximately a quarter of respondents argued that, although it is of fundamental importance, nurses have some way to go before they can fully support individuals with cancer, as they are not educated to deal with this role effectively. Thus, several respondents argued that the potential is enormous:

> *It is probably the most important thing that could be done although it isn't always done.*
>
> *(cf category F1.2)*

Only 33% of respondents, similar to the literature (see p41), commented on their lack of education in psychosocial aspects of care. However, several respondents expressed their feelings of inadequacy and frustration:

> *At times you do feel useless when you know that there is nothing else you can do... it's when you know that you can't do anything... if somebody just rejects you and just won't let you get really close.*
>
> *I myself feel fairly inadequate with some of the patients... it's just sometimes they ask for you... and really I have no idea how to answer them... I go and ask someone else.*
>
> *(cf category F1.2)*

Thirty-three per cent of respondents stated that they wanted more training in this area, in order to carry out their support role effectively. For example:

> *More training would be helpful to know how to recognise stress and how to deal with it, how to counsel patients.*
>
> *...with stress there are no 'hard and fast' guidelines or set list of indicators and not everyone observes the same things, thus we need more guidance.*
>
> *We need the availability of study days as often we're so busy you may miss a lot of stress factors in the patient.*
>
> *(cf category G3)*

(This relates directly to theme 12 regarding methods of helping nurses assess stress in persons with cancer.)

Only 25% of respondents commented on their need for support, in keeping with the literature (see p41). These respondents spoke of the need for support groups, in order for them to, in turn, effectively support persons with cancer. For example:

> *There is a need for a wider, larger support group so that everybody is in a position to talk about their problems, the problem with this is the size of the people involved.*
>
> *Support groups for staff would ultimately help us help the patients.*
>
> *(cf category G3)*

A significant minority of respondents (18%) stated the central importance of experience in relation to assessing stress in persons with cancer. They explained that they learned from watching and discussing with experienced fellow staff:

> *I think a lot of it comes through experience... watching your seniors — or sometimes an auxiliary... a lot of it is experience and maturity really.*
>
> *...just experience is the best way... sharing things that you do sort out and things people told you with other people.*
>
> *...a lot of it is just through experience... through talking to people that have been here obviously a lot longer.*
>
> *You can be taught skills, but not everybody can do it... it's just experience...*
>
> *(cf category G2)*

However, it is important to consider the quality of the experience gained, otherwise, as Bond (1982) states, experience in communication is often gained in an *ad hoc* manner with possible adverse effects. For example, staff may easily and unwittingly learn closed forms of communication from inappropriate role models, which would actively hinder open patterns of communication with persons with cancer.

Eighteen per cent of respondents suggested the use of an instrument to help nurses assess psychosocial aspects of a person's care. For example:

> *...a tool similar to a pain assessment chart would be useful to see how a patient progresses... if we can do this with pain, why not with stress which is also important?*
>
> *To develop a simple tool to incorporate into the care plan that will actually allow you to make decisions regarding areas causing stress.*
>
> *To be aware of what areas might be stressed and to have them jotted down or consigned to memory might just make you look out for different things...*
>
> *(cf category G4)*

They also acknowledged the importance of discussion of these areas with other health care professionals:

> *...instead of normal ward routines, to involve people like Macmillan nurses and have 'ward rounds' in the office and talk about patients and how they thought they were coping.*

> *It's most important to be able to talk with colleagues about a patient and achieve something constructive regarding future change... it's having the opportunity to bring stress onto the agenda.*

> *(cf category G3)*

To conclude, themes 10 and 12 illustrate the fragmentation present within the interview findings, which are indicative of a phenomenological perspective. Although all respondents discussed their support role, a consistent picture did not emerge. For example, the mis-match present between 33% of respondents who emphasised the value of more educational initiatives and 18% of respondents who valued the central role of experience. This fragmentation reflects the common-sense knowledge of the respondents which is derived largely from their individual professional and vocational experiences, as well as from education.

Theme 11: nursing respondents' views regarding the nursing process

When asked regarding modes of communication, 80% of respondents spoke of the importance of verbal forms of communication:

> *It is more immediate and not open to interpretation thus the message is clearer and easier to use.*

> *You can find out more about patients from the rest of the team.*

> *Quite often it's something that you can't actually pinpoint so I usually talk to whoever is in charge.*

> *...able to give much more information verbally.*

> *(cf category G1)*

When asked directly regarding the nursing process, 73% of respondents spoke of the problems associated with it. It is encouraging that it was not the nursing process *per se* that was problematic, rather it was the widely held view that the nursing Kardex was not being used effectively. For example:

It is not used for stress but more for basic nursing care.

You don't always look in the Kardex... so no point recording it if it's never to be read again.

It's not always read by staff or updated regularly.

It's often done automatically, not really thought about... for example anxiety is often written as a main problem and set responses to suit.

(cf category G1.1)

Seventy-five per cent of respondents confirmed the author's own experience that the Kardex was not used for psychosocial aspects of a person's care. They noted that the format was inadequate, due to its emphasis on physiological aspects of care. These respondents also reflected observations that the actual presentation and layout of the Kardex made it extremely difficult for the nurse to record a concise psychosocial assessment, which could then be easily seen and read by other members of the health care team:

It is difficult to see progression of a patient's psychological state in the progress notes as you don't have the time to go back and read through all the pages... if you've been off, it's difficult to tell from that where a patient has got to.

With the current Kardex, significant conversations with a patient frequently get overlooked by nurses as there is not a special place in the Kardex for details to be recorded.

(cf category G1.1)

Several respondents admitted that there were problems related to lack of knowledge on how to use the nursing Kardex properly:

I don't think it's used properly anyway, I don't think anybody knows fully how to implement the nursing process... people... just rely on the ward report and then obviously sometimes it's just by fate that you come across things.

It's difficult to write down about stress unless it's a long-winded affair and the whole point of the nursing process is that it is something which is done quickly.

It's difficult to write down about a patient's problem... there are problems sometimes of confidentiality with recorded information.

(cf category G1.1)

Several respondents also raised significant issues regarding the use of the nursing Kardex. For example, does it make any difference to patient care at the end of the day?

It doesn't appear to make a vast improvement to people's mental state by writing an additional problem in their Kardex.

(cf category G1.1)

However, it is encouraging that 80% of respondents saw positive aspects of nursing Kardex:

Good to have guidelines.

More continuity — everyone knows what has been said if a conversation has been recorded.

Verbal information can get lost, especially if someone has days off.

We are all human at the end of the day.

If you haven't nursed an individual before, it helps to look in the Kardex and see problems so you're aware of them.

The information is readily available.

The information you can get out of them is good... if you are worried, to fall back on it.

...able to evaluate care by use of the nursing process.

(cf category G1.1)

Several respondents made positive suggestions, as they recommended recording the information given regarding the person's cancer diagnosis and prognosis and also perceptions of stress.

To conclude, although 80% of respondents acknowledged and discussed the current problems associated with the ineffective use of the Kardex, they were also able to argue the positive aspects of its effective use.

Conclusion — themes

It can be seen from these twelve themes that two disparate philosophies emerge. First, the biomedical model is in evidence in themes 1 and 2 which deal with the negative attitudes surrounding cancer and in theme 6 which covers treatment and its side effects, and key indicators of stress. In contrast, a humanistic approach, reflective of a broad phenomenological approach, is prevalent in theme 3 (the family), theme 4 (helplessness), theme 5 (effect of cancer on lifestyle and theme 8 (pain and analgesia). However, within several themes (e.g. theme 7 on altered body image and theme 9 on coping and coping patterns) both contrasting philosophies were present, which indicates the complex nature of the views of nursing staff regarding stress and the person with cancer.

Content analysis — observations

The development of key categories

Five broad category systems were developed which focus on persons with cancer. In keeping with previous research findings, the categories predominantly reflect the significant areas of omission by the majority of nursing respondents in relation to stress and persons with cancer (see p40). Some categories were also discerned from individuals' non-verbal responses to situations, as observed by the researcher, and from their own verbal responses to the areas raised by the nurses (or, on several occasions raised by themselves). The five category systems are shown in Tables 9.11, 9.12, 9.13, 9.14 and 9.15.

The frequency table, Table 9.16, highlights the key similarities and differences amongst the thirty nurses, who each carried out an admission assessment, in terms of their communication patterns, the main psychological areas raised, significant omissions and overall references to physiological and psychological factors.

Table 9.11 H categories: patient's psychological state

category H1	patient able to express psychological state
category H1.1	brief statement affirming satisfactory psychological state
category H1.2	verbal references to anxiety
category H1.3	non-verbal cues regarding anxiety
category H2	patient expresses psychological state in physiological terms
category H3	patient initiated communication
category H3.1	patient controlled communication

Table 9.12 I categories: patient's concerns at present time

category I1	patient able to express concerns
category I1.1	brief statment regarding lack of concerns
category I2	concern to get better
category I2.1	concern regarding future outlook
category I2.2	concern to return to 'normal' lifestyle
category I3	concern about change of lifestyle
category I3.1	concern about effect on work
category I4	concern about significant others
category I5	concern about being alone at home
category I6	concern about pain
category I7	concern about hospitalisation and/or hospital staff
category I8	concern about treatment and its side effects
category I8.1	concern about loss of hair
category I8.2	concern about nausea

Table 9.13 J categories: patient's perception of illness and treatment

category J1	patient able to mention word 'cancer'
category J1.1	patient's perceptions of cancer
category J1.2	patient's use of euphemisms
category J1.3	patient's use of medical terminology
category J2	patient able to explain nature of his/her illness
category J2.1	patient gives vague explanation of his/her illness
category J3	patient aware of nature of treatment
category J3.1	patient unaware of nature of treatment
category J4	patient able to explain information given by consultant regarding his/her illness and/or treatment
category J4.1	patient refers to state of his/her memory
category J5	patient able to give details of his/her medical history

Table 9.14 K categories: patient's coping mechanisms

category K1	patient able to verbalise regarding his/her coping mechanisms
category K2	references to patient blocking illness at present time
category K3	references to adjusting to illness
category K4	references to use of emotions
category K5	references to fighting illness
category K6	references to religious beliefs/use of prayer
category K7	references to faith in medical staff

Table 9.15 L categories: patient's support network

category L1	patient perceives family to be supportive
category L1.1	lack of family support
category L2	patient able to communicate openly with family regarding his/her concerns
category L2.1	lack of open communication with family
category L3	family able to give patient practical support
category L4	patient perceives extended support network (e.g. friends, distant relatives, social services) to be supportive
category L4.1	lack of an extended support network
category L5	patient able to communicate openly with extended support network regarding his/her concerns
category L5.1	lack of open communication with extended support network
category L6	extended support network able to give patient practical support

Key areas explored by nursing respondents and significant omissions

The phenomenological approach was used in order to analyse the key similarities and differences amongst nurses, in relation to their respective nursing admission assessments. The rationale behind this being that verbal and non-verbal cues are likely to influence the responses of a person with cancer, in relation to his/her perceptions of stress. The observation findings, similar to the interview findings, are examined in conjunction with the relevant literature, in order to

Table 9.16 Frequency of responses from nurse respondents

Response	Number
open style communication	21
closed style communication	7
use of elaborations/probes	14
use of blocking tactics	7
initiated communication	18
controlled communication	14
equal communication	15
use of positive non-verbal communication	24

key psychological areas:
    current concerns
    perceptions of illness
    family and social circumstances
	
	23
	26
	21

significant omissions:
    psychological state
    perception of treatment
    reaction to hospitalisation
    reaction to hospital itself
    coping patterns
    communication with family (significant others) regarding
      concerns (including diagnosis)
	
	21
	21
	17
	29
	29
	29

overall psychological orientation	**14**
overall psychosocial orientation	**3**
equal orientation	**13**

information giving:
    physiological aspects (including treatment)
    psychosocial areas (e.g. ward layout)
	
	22
	10

note taking	**16**

create a firm theoretical framework for the assessment of stress, as applied to the person with cancer.

Overall, the nurses fared better than their counterparts in previous research findings on communication and psychosocial aspects of care (see p40). In terms of the dynamics of the patterns of communication, 70% adopted an open style of communication and, to further support this, 80% used positive non-verbal communication. There were also very few overt blocking tactics employed (23%), in contrast to the findings of Bond (1982).

Although 46% controlled the communication, 50% allowed the person with cancer equal control of the communication. These findings are encouraging and are more positive than the earlier research findings of Bond (1982) and Maguire (1985) (see p40).

However, there is still room for significant improvement regarding communication patterns, as only 46% made use of elaboration cues. Despite 76% asking an open question regarding the concerns of the person with cancer, only 46% followed this through with probing to further explore any possible psychosocial problems or needs. As a result, 53% of individuals with cancer outlined their main concerns. An overall picture was gained. Thirty-three per cent highlighted physiologically-based concerns. For example:

Pain

> *I can't remember walking without pain... not since I've been in hospital.*

> *I wish I could get comfortable.*

> *(cf category I6)*

(From the researcher's observation notes: The individual commented that he had not received any analgesia since 6.30a.m. He was usually taking oral Diamorphine. The time of the interview was 4.00pm.)

Treatment and its side effects

> *I'm worried about the treatment making me feel sick... drips worry me.*

> *(cf category I8.2)*

> *The treatment worries me... I must go through with it.*

> *...I was terribly ill after the treatment...*

> *(cf category I8)*

Thirty per cent of individuals outlined concerns relating to psychosocial aspects of their illness:

Concerns to return to normal lifestyle

> *I want to get it all done and get back to a fairly normal life.*

> *(cf category I2.2)*

Concern regarding family

I wake up worrying about my husband.

(cf category I4)

Concern regarding the illness and the future

At times it hits you... where's it going to end?... I just keep wondering if it's going to work.

(cf category I2.1)

No, no, no... don't you think I've told you enough... everything's wrong with me...

(Observation notes: The person was angry and subsequently burst into tears (cf category I2.1)).

The lack of any detailed exploration by 54% of nurses reflects Maguire's findings (1985b), that nurses often fail to clarify the responses of a person with cancer.

As regards the key psychosocial areas explored by the nurses, the results, on the surface, appear more positive than previous research findings. This is largely due to the fact that 80% of the nurses explored the person's perceptions of his/her illness. Fifty per cent of persons with cancer were able to give details of their medical history. Thirty-seven per cent were unable to explain the exact nature of their illness. For example, one person explained that he was involved in a serious road traffic accident and whilst on back rest in hospital, he started having 'water works' trouble. He explained that they found 'two warts in bladder', 'said growth there... take it out by radium treatment and hopefully it will do the trick...' When asked about the growth the person replied, 'Yes, cancer' (cf category J2).

Thirty seven per cent of persons with cancer mentioned the word 'cancer' during their explanation of their illness:

I think it's a kind of cancer... I'm waiting to get some treatment going...

(cf category J1)

Vague explanations regarding the nature of their illness, were given by 37% of persons with cancer, revealing their partial denial of the exact cause of the illness and its implications. For example:

I've never had anything the matter with me before... what's on my bladder... I think it's an ulcer...

(cf category J2.1)

Thirty-seven per cent of persons with cancer made use of euphemisms for the word 'cancer'. (NB it was not possible to determine from the interviews whether the medical staff had first made use of a euphemism or whether the person had chosen to use one.) The following terms were used:

'growth'; 'tumour', 'wart'; 'ulcer'; 'lump'; 'lesion'.

During their respective interviews, 20% of individuals with cancer denied the nature of their illness. For example:

> *I've had my breast off... I don't know what's wrong with me... my bust and that must be all right...*

(cf category J2.1)

Forty-three per cent of individuals were able to recall the information given to them by the consultant. However, it was not possible to determine from the admission assessment the exact information given to the person by the consultant. Thus, it was not possible to explore whether the person recalled all the information accurately or not. When asked about their perceptions of their illness, 13% of persons with cancer referred to the state of their memory. One person admitted:

> *I've a rotten memory... I can't remember what he said... put something in my womb... 100% curable... I can't remember.*

(cf category J4.1)

Similar to the high percentage of nurses who explored persons' perceptions of their illness, 70% explored the person's support network, albeit mainly in terms of practical support. In reply, 53% of persons with cancer gave brief details regarding their family members and stated that they were well. Thirteen per cent of individuals with cancer admitted that their family had ill health and that they were concerned for them. For example, one person explained that both her parents had had strokes:

> *I can't help them very much... they have a home help. I take them shopping. I do worry... only my husband is left... my mum worried about me... I've got to be very careful... there's nobody else to do it.*

(cf category I4)

Thirty-seven per cent of persons with cancer gave brief details of where they lived and explained that their significant others, relatives or neighbours were supportive. For example:

I have three nieces, one of which I looked after when she was three months old, now she does everything for me.

(cf category L1)

Seventeen per cent of persons with cancer gave implicit references to their concern regarding their present or future ability to manage in their home. For example, one person who had recently moved to a new bungalow admitted that she had had a:

...slight fall in the bathroom... my husband lost his grasp.

(cf category I2.1)

When asked about their home circumstances, 6% of individuals gave implicit references to their social isolation. One person explained that she was completely on her own and 'very rarely' saw her cousin and 'relied on neighbours' for her shopping.

However, there were many significant omissions, which support the earlier findings of Bond (1982), that nurses tend to give a low level of attention to psychosocial aspects of a person's illness (see p41). It was surprising that very few nurses (approximately 3-5%) explored all key psychosocial areas, as all the nurses were aware of the nature of the study. To their credit, they were not biased by the study and carried out the admission assessment as in their everyday practice. As a result, a person's psychological state was only explored by 30% of nurses.

Individuals with cancer who were asked directly, explained their psychological state using physiological indicators:

...terrible... I feel rotten all over... I can't even walk.

I have lost weight with worrying... I find if difficult to relax... I was so relieved at the treatment... it's not so bad as I thought.

(cf category H2)

When asked directly, 13% of persons with cancer made brief affirmative statements that they were all right. For example:

I feel OK...

...not so bad now...

(cf category H1.1)

Very few nurses picked up on the non-verbal cues of persons with cancer in relation to anxiety. The researcher detected overt signs of anxiety in 24 persons. For example, from the observation notes: rubbing hands together frequently; occasional eye contact with the nurse; looked down frequently; touched ear frequently; spoke very quickly; use of 'er', 'um' and 'ah hah'; small frequent smiles; touched face frequently; folded arms frequently; lack of eye contact with the nurse; frequent head nodding; laughed quickly when making a joke; frequently touched housecoat; undoing and fastening the buttons of the housecoat; losing track of words he/she wished to express. Most individuals made use of several of these cues, which substantiated their explicit and implicit references to their anxiety.

For those persons with cancer who gave implicit verbal references, the non-verbal cues of anxiety substantiated the researcher's observation notes regarding the individuals' psychological state during their admission assessments. For example:

Patient appeared very anxious — she spoke very quickly and voiced her fear of the paracentesis and her worry regarding her family — she appeared to almost break down but trailed off mid-sentence.

Patient appeared extremely anxious, stopped and trailed off mid-sentence — looked down at nurse's notes or straight in front of him... patient associated start of his trouble with picking up something heavy... patient spoke in mainly monosyllables.

This reflects Bond's findings (1982) that nurses often ignore cues regarding a person's psychological state. Although 32% of nurses revealed their awareness of non-verbal communication and gave clear examples during the interviews with the researcher, they did not subsequently appear to actively use this knowledge during the admission assessments of those persons with cancer who revealed overt anxiety cues. As Lazarus argues (1966), people undervalue non-verbal means of communication and, therefore, are missing influential messages.

The person's perceptions regarding treatment were only explored by 30% of the nurses. In reply, 13% of persons gave brief explanations of the nature of their treatment:

...deep x-rays... shrink or stop its growth altogether.

...take growth out by radium treatment and, hopefully, it will do the trick.

(cf category J3)

An individual's coping patterns were ignored by 97% of nurses. This reflects Maguire *et al*'s findings (1980a) that the majority of nurses do not routinely inquire regarding a person's psychosocial adjustment (see p40). Thirty percent of persons gave implicit verbal references of ways of coping during their respective interviews, which were not detected by the nurses. Fifteen per cent of persons with cancer gave references to coping via adopting a fighting spirit regarding their lives. For example:

> *You've got to be positive... you can't give in. I'd feel happier if there was a 100% cure, but they won't give you that... I've got lots of things to be positive about... I want to get it all done and get back to a fairly normal life... I'm not thinking of the treatment lasting till November... I'm taking it each one at a time... when I've had three, I'll be half way through.*

(cf category K5)

An individual with cancer referred to his religious beliefs. He mentioned his Catholic faith and stated, 'this and my family will help me cope with my illness.' A respondent referred to adjusting to the diagnosis of cancer:

> *I've steadied down... I packed in my job... I'm comfy in my own house... I've had nerve tablets... I don't enjoy going out... lost confidence — due to breathing... I find it difficult to relax... I can manage things... I think these things come... it hit me all at once... I know my limits now...*

(cf category K3)

Another respondent referred to blocking out their illness at present:

> *I'll just take it as it comes... just trying to blot it out really... I don't talk about it to anybody... I hide it...*

(cf category K2)

An individual revealed that expressing emotions acted as a means of coping. For example, from the observation notes: one person explained that she cried when she had a dilatation and curettage and she later broke down and cried in the interview when she stated she had cancer.

Only 56% of nurses asked persons directly about their reaction to hospitalisation, in response to which 23% of persons with cancer spoke of their concern. For example:

> *I've only been in hospital once six years ago, then at X... I'm not frightened since I've been in there... as long as I get better.*

(cf category I7)

Ten per cent of persons with cancer, when asked, were non-committal and did not reveal their reaction to hospitalisation. Hospitalisation was regarded in a positive light by 6% of individuals:

> *I'm hoping they can ease it [pain] off a bit...*
>
> *(cf category I7)*

Only one nurse asked directly regarding the person's reaction to the hospital itself. Similarly, with regard to the person's support network, only one nurse full explored the family communication patterns about concerns. For example, when the nurse asked a person whether her husband was fully aware of her illness and whether he understood, she replied:

> *No... just about radiotherapy... just trying to blot it out really... I don't talk about it... I hide it...*
>
> *(cf category L2.1)*

Thus, three key psychosocial areas were not explored by 97% of nurses during respective admission interviews: reaction to hospital itself; coping patterns; communication with family regarding concerns. These findings reflect the professional bias recognised by Bond (1982) (see p41) towards the physiological symptoms of a person's illness. Thus, 46% of nurses had an overall physiological orientation and only 10% had an overriding psychosocial orientation. However, it is encouraging to note that 43% of nurses had an equal orientation during the respective interviews.

Concerning information giving, it is encouraging that all nurses gave the person information. However, 73% of nurses focused solely on physiological aspects of the illness, including treatment. Only 33% in contrast, gave information relating to psychosocial aspects of illness (e.g. ward layout and routine, which previous research suggests is important, in order to reduce a person's stress). These figures relate to the implications from previous research (see p42), that persons with cancer are generally dissatisfied with the quality of information they receive.

The observation data supports the previous arguments put forward by Maguire (1985b), and it appears that a significant number of nurses are still maintaining an emotional distance from persons with cancer. As Maguire suggests, these nurses are worried that raising psychosocial areas may lead to difficult questions, increased workload and additional stress for themselves. Clearly, all the nurses acknowledged these problems in their interviews with the researcher.

Indeed, 33% of nurses argued that, in order to address these psychosocial areas, they need adequate training. Unfortunately, as argued by Maguire (1978), the ultimate implication remains that persons with cancer are failing to receive the psychological support they need and their perceptions of stress may easily be exacerbated as a direct result of this.

To conclude, it can be seen that the observation categories reveal the common-sense worlds of the nursing respondents, in relation to the nursing admission assessments carried out with individuals with cancer. Therefore, the nurses' interpretations are based on their knowledge and understanding of the situation which, in turn, is influenced by their experiences and their training. The categories also reveal the direct effects of the areas covered (or not) by the nurses, in relation to an individual's perceptions of stress. As a result, the biomedical model is much more in evidence in the observation findings than in the interview findings, due to the significant areas of omission relating to psychosocial aspects of care (e.g. an individual's psychological state and coping patterns). The observation findings parallel the literature with regard to patients' concerns and the support role of the nurse. Thus, these observation findings contribute to the body of knowledge regarding stress and the person with cancer.

Content analysis — archival sources

Key areas recorded and significant omissions by the nursing respondents

An examination of 20 nursing Kardexes was carried out (n=20), to explore if any discrepancies existed regarding the recorded information from the nursing admission assessment, in relation to psychosocial aspects of care. The archival courses acted as a useful crosschecking method and, therefore, as a means of validating the data gained in the other areas of the study.

There was a lack of documentation regarding psychosocial aspects of a person's care, which reflected the problem highlighted by 73% of nurses in the interviews, i.e. that the nursing Kardex was not used properly in many cases (see p128). This also endorses the literature regarding the lack of documentation recording a person's pain (see p62). In contrast to the suggestions of the previous literature, the presence of a person (in this case, the researcher) at the time information was recorded on the Kardex, did not make the process of retrieving this information any easier. As a result, aspects relating to psychosocial dimensions of a person's illness were significant by their absence.

However, there were several key areas that were briefly recorded, which largely reflected the areas explored by the nurses in respective admission assessments. The person's perceptions of their illness were recorded in approximately one sentence in 17 out of 20 Kardexes. For example:

Knows he has 'chest cancer' diagnosed Xmas 1987.

Patient knows he had a malignant tumour of his bone. He is having chemo now as a precautionary measure to clear any stray cells.

It is probable, as argued by 73% of nurses in their interviews with the researcher (see p130), that the current format dictates the lack of adequate reporting of psychosocial aspects of a person's care. This is due to the fact that, in the Kardex of the hospital concerned, there are only three lines reserved to record a patient's perceptions of his/her illness.

A person's reaction to hospitalisation was briefly recorded in 15 out of 20 Kardexes. For example:

Not unduly anxious.

Obviously concerned.

Resigned.

The small space allocated encourages the use of a standardised question, but this is not followed through with any relevant substantiating information. Eight Kardexes reported individuals as having positive reactions to hospitalisation, similar to the research interview findings in which nurses acknowledged the possible positive effects. However, due to the lack of supporting information and the large number of persons with cancer that the researcher observed as revealing overt anxiety cues (80%), the validity of these reports are questionable. Only four Kardexes recorded a negative reaction to hospitalisation. As found in the admission assessments, the majority of nurses were not fully aware of the person's cues and subsequently they were not recorded in the Kardex.

The majority of notes regarding social circumstances (in 18 out of 20 Kardexes) reflect the emphasis on practical matters by the respective nurse during the admission assessments. Most notes recorded information regarding where the person lived and brief details regarding their family and social services, location of bathroom etc, as appropriate:

> *Lives with wife who is in good health at present. No problems which may affect discharge.*

> *Lives in detached house. Toilet and bathroom facilities upstairs. Husband is presently suffering from pre-senile dementia — is going to see Dr X at C on Wed. J does not foresee any problems on discharge at present — aware of MSW if needed. Two daughters — both nearby.*

The effects of the disease on a person's activities of daily living (ADLs) was recorded in 16 out of 20 Kardexes and mainly covered physiological aspects of a person's illness. For example: elimination; diet; mobility; pain; breathing; appetite; sleep; maintaining a safe environment; personal cleansing and dressing.

This clearly reflects the physiological orientation of nearly half of the nursing admission assessments and also highlights the prime concern of the nurse as reported in the previous literature.

With regard to a person's psychological state, although this was not explored directly in the respective admission assessments, nine Kardexes referred to it. Seven referred to the person's anxiety, which reflects the literature that cues are often missed, as the researcher detected anxiety cues in 80% of persons with cancer. For example:

> *Very anxious — particularly about being sick.*

> *Quiet, anxious man admitted for lymphoma workup.*

Of the seven brief statements regarding persons' physiological state, only three followed the problem through to the care plan.

There were also clear contradictions present, as six Kardexes recorded anxiety as a problem in the care plan, despite an earlier statement that the person's psychological state was satisfactory or was not previously recorded. This reflects the tendency, acknowledged by several nurses in the interviews, to automatically record anxiety as a problem with routine nursing actions underneath, without due consideration to the individual concerned and his/her particular situation. Evidently, the care plan easily becomes meaningless. Nurses need to ensure that individuals' psychosocial states are carefully assessed and that the prevalent standardisation of persons' needs and problems is avoided.

The progress notes revealed sparse information regarding a person's psychosocial well-being, which reflects the lack of exploration in the admission assessment regarding a person's psychological state. Similar to the routine use of the word 'anxiety' in the care plans, there was frequent use of the term 'has settled on to the ward', which lacks meaning in itself. For example:

Appears to have settled on to the ward.

Appears to have settled reasonably well, finding it hard not being quite so active.

No complaints identified this pm.

As previously argued in the literature (see p41), this reflects the lack of education regarding psychological forms of patient assessment and effective documentation.

Another significant omission, which reflects the observation findings, is references to coping. There were no references to coping in any of the Kardexes. The lack of a specific heading within the Kardex does not encourage exploration of this area. There were no references to interaction with a person's family regarding his/her illness, or to referrals made to other health care professionals, despite both having separate space to document this information.

Although 73% of nurses gave information to respective persons with cancer about the physiological aspects of their illness and treatment, only one Kardex recorded the information given. As a result, in all other cases, members of staff could not be aware of exactly what the persons with cancer had been told, without verbally asking the nurse or person concerned. This could easily lead to repetitive information giving on an *ad hoc* basis, instead of information being carefully geared to the individual. This reflects the literature's criticisms of information-giving by nursing staff. It is also in keeping with the research interview findings, as the lack of recorded information suggests that nurses tend to rely on verbal means of communication. The resultant problem with this is that key information relating to a person's psychosocial welfare may not be passed on to relevant staff and the person's family.

To conclude, the sparse and often routine recording of psychosocial information reflects the inadequate assessment of a person's psychosocial state on admission to hospital. In keeping with the interview and observation findings, and the relevant literature, this points to an urgent need for education regarding psychosocial aspects of care. The archival sources also reveal that the nursing Kardex is not used as an integral form of communication, despite the majority of nurses being aware of its advantages.

10 Discussion of principle findings of the study and recommendations

Interview findings

A discussion of the differences amongst nurses from the interview data regarding their key philosophies in relation to stress amongst persons with cancer

It can be seen in Chapter 9 that, in accordance with a phenomenological approach, the everyday world of the nurses reveals a rich diversity and depth of information. Emerging from the data are two disparate views regarding stress and persons with cancer: a biomedical approach and a humanistic approach. It is not straightforward enough to propose that 'x' number of nurses hold a medical model view and 'y' number hold a humanistic model view. Rather, the views of the cancer nurses vary according to the subject raised. It is much more likely that there exists a mixture of these philosophies amongst the nurses, which reflects the nature of their personal everyday experiences and the nature of their education.

Within the death theme (theme 1) of the interviews, the biomedical model is the prevalent underlying philosophy. There is a strong sense of the all encompassing negative attitudes of cancer being synonymous with death, dying and suffering, due to the lack of an overall medical cure. This reflects the dominant influence of the philosophy of biomedicine and its cure-oriented basis, as opposed to a clear emphasis on a caring approach and the quality of life. The nature of nurses' pre- and post-registration training is also reflected, i.e. the biomedical emphasis on the pathophysiology of cancer and its treatment. Nurses' everyday experiences are mirrored, as it is probable that, through their experience, they hold the common assumption that all the patients on the cancer ward will die at some point. Hence, the focus is likely to rest on the number of individuals with cancer who have died, as opposed to the individual's quality of life right up until the terminal stages of the illness.

The power of the biomedical model is further evident in the treatment theme (theme 6), due to the mainstream acceptance of treating cancer with westernised medicine, which takes the form of complex regimes of cytotoxic chemotherapy and radiotherapy. Most nurses focused on the problems of nausea and vomiting. They adopted a biomedical approach to chemophobia by outlining the key stimuli responsible. In contrast to a humanistic approach, they failed to explore the role of anxiety on individuals with cancer, or to acknowledge the complex nature of anticipatory nausea and vomiting. A quarter of nurses reflected a medical approach with respect to the effects of alopecia. They normalised the problems associated with alopecia and argued that persons with cancer were more concerned with saving their lives. Again, the emphasis was placed on a curative rather than a caring approach.

However, a mismatch of beliefs is evident here, which reflects the complexity of the data and belies the simplistic notion that a certain number of nurses hold a particular philosophy. In contrast to the above, over half of the nurses reflected a humanistic approach, as they acknowledged the problems associated with alopecia and substantiated their views with examples from their everyday clinical experiences. Thus, despite the overall biomedical influence regarding cancer equalling death, approximately half of the nurses were able to reflect on experiences with patients, which contradicted the medical notion of the normalisation of the side-effects of treatment. In this way, their experiences, with regard to the effects of alopecia, helped to develop a humanistic approach in keeping with more recent nursing literature.

A humanistic approach was equally apparent within the family theme (theme 3), probably due to the emotive nature of the family. A quarter of the nurses gave vivid examples from their everyday work experiences of the stress experienced by mothers, regarding the well-being of their children. These nurses reacted emotionally, by giving examples which they judged to be important in terms of meaning for themselves. The majority of the nurse respondents gave specific examples of the effects of cancer on partner relationships. In keeping with a phenomenological approach, the nurses reflected the influences of their own particular situations. This acts in sharp contrast to a detached medical stance, which does not often give primary value to personal feelings, and it is probable that nurses subconsciously dismissed a biomedical model as inappropriate, due to the complex emotions involved in the family theme.

Similarly, there were a significant number of nurses who adopted a humanistic approach within the helplessness theme (theme 4), as they acknowledged the importance of a perceived lack of control, i.e. the role of psychological factors, as opposed to actual loss of control in solely physiological terms.

Within the lifestyle theme (theme 5), a quarter of nurses gave specific examples regarding the loss of plans for the future. This linked to the family theme (theme 3), as these nurses, in keeping with a phenomenological approach, were giving examples of individuals they had nursed in their everyday work experience. Also similar to the family theme, nurses provided examples which probably held a central meaning and importance for themselves. In a sense, the nurses were not only drawing from the reality of the hospital ward, but were possibly subconsciously role-playing the significance of these events, with the question 'What would happen if it were me?' in mind. It is a question concerning the cancer nurse, but one that the cancer nurse would not readily ask of him/herself. However, once it has arisen, it cannot easily be ignored and demands an answer, which at once reveals the fragility and vulnerability of human nature.

A humanistic approach is also highlighted by half of the nurses within the altered body image theme (theme 7), regarding the effects of surgical disfigurement. These nurses explored the psychological effects of mastectomy on individuals and the individuals' relationships with their partners. This area probably reflects the implicit concerns of the nurses, the majority of whom are women, as the subject of mastectomy is an emotive issue for women in western society. It can be seen that a significant proportion of nurses in the interviews made use of their common-sense understandings of their daily work experiences and personal situations, to give a greater insight into the psychological stress of persons with cancer.

It is not suggested that a humanistic approach is reflected by a significant proportion of the nurses throughout the key themes. This notion is too simplistic, as the biomedical approach has been seen to be prevalent in an all pervading sense with the death, stigma and treatment themes (themes 1, 2 and 6). Within the altered body image theme, there is a noticeable absence of exploration regarding the psychological effects of cancer on an individual's sexuality. Despite the growing nursing literature on this subject in relation to the key role of the nurse, the lack of discussion by nurses is probably a reflection of the biomedical emphasis (to the exclusion of complex human and moral issues) in their training.

In keeping with a curative approach, it could be argued that the nurses did not regard issues of sexuality to be of central importance, in comparison with life and death issues and the family. Equally, it could be argued that, in accordance with a medical approach, the subject of sexuality is considered a taboo subject and does not readily warrant discussion, unless an individual discloses a severe sexual problem meriting psychiatric intervention. This is in direct contrast to a humanistic approach, which moves away from problem identification to promotion of sexual health, in which an exploration of a person's perceptions of sexuality are essential.

The fragmentation present within the interview findings in relation to the two opposing philosophies is highlighted in relation to indicators of stress. Initially, a humanistic approach is evident, as nearly half of the nurses acknowledged the importance of knowing an individual, in order to assess their perceptions of stress. Similarly, a quarter of the nurses discussed their intuitive feelings regarding individuals. However, most nurses simultaneously reflected a biomedical approach, as they discussed the role of behavioural factors which were based on generalisations and stereotypes of persons with cancer, as opposed to specific individuals. Half of the nurses also explained the importance of physiological indicators of stress, clearly highlighting the focus of Selye's response-based model and in keeping with a biomedical model. These contrasting philosophies appear to run almost parallel to one another. At times, the biomedical approach appears to take the lead, and at others a humanistic model emerges as the dominant philosophy.

This becomes much more apparent when the nurses turned to the subject of coping. Their overall views clearly reflected a biomedical model, as they conveyed a judgmental approach regarding the most 'effective' patterns of coping (e.g. the person with cancer having a positive outlook and a 'fighting spirit'). This carries the notion that there is a 'preferred' way of coping, as the individual who adopts these coping patterns is much more amenable to health care professionals than someone who is withdrawn or who denies his/her illness. In this judgmental approach, the health care professional dons the role of the expert and assumes for others (i.e. individuals with cancer) the 'acceptable' forms of coping. This reflects the medical tradition of health care professionals having greater power than the lay person, and is in sharp contrast to a humanistic approach, in which the individual is the expert regarding all matters that concern the self.

However, when the nurses explored the subject of coping in greater detail, a very different approach was revealed. Nearly half of the nurses emphasised the importance of knowing the individual in order to assess how he/she is coping. Three quarters of the nurses acknowledged that individuals cope in different ways and the nurses were able to give examples relating to specific individuals they had nursed. Both these points reflect a humanistic perspective. It is possible that the nurses were not as overtly aware of these views as of those views indicative of a biomedical model. Instead, a humanistic approach appears to lie beneath the surface of the nurse's consciousness. This is probably due to the prevalent influence of the medical model in cancer nursing, stemming from the medical treatments given to persons with cancer and the subsequently ensuing power of the consultant oncologists, physicians and radiotherapists.

In keeping with a humanistic approach, all the nurses acknowledged the centrality of the support role of the cancer nurse and a third of the nurses openly commented on their need for further training in psychosocial aspects of care. Could it be the influence of the recent nursing press, regarding psychological aspects of care, and the increase in the number of national and regional conferences, study days and short courses that have led to this awareness? Or, conversely, do the nurses make use of their common-sense understandings of their role and emphathetically intuit that psychological support should play a key part in the care of the persons with cancer? (That is, from their experiences of caring for persons with cancer, the cancer nurses respond as human beings to fellow human beings and perceive the importance of psychological care.)

These arguments provide a simplistic explanation. It is much more likely that the cancer nurse's caring qualities are eroded by the mainstream prime concern with the medicalisation of the person with cancer. In addition, the situational constraints (e.g ward organisation, staffing numbers and skill mix, workload) explained by several nurses, divert the attention of the cancer nurse away from his/her support role. Also, as previously argued in the literature, the cancer nurse does not always naturally acquire the communication skills required to carry out a support role. The nurse may learn these skills from a poor role model (i.e. a fellow nurse) on an *ad hoc* basis in the ward situation. Thus, the type of training the nurse has experienced is also a significant factor to consider.

At present, the educational experiences of cancer nurses are varied. As previously argued, there still remains a dominant medical influence, due to the prevalence of medical treatments being used to treat cancer. It is likely that qualified nurses have spent a much smaller proportion of time during their registered general nurse training, on psychosocial aspects of care in comparison to physical care. Even for those nurses who have completed the oncology course certified by the English National Board, the majority of courses offered at regional centres (with one notable exception) still reflect the physiologically-based focus of care for persons with cancer. It is likely that it will take a significant period of time before the psychological needs of person with cancer are taken on board. Recently, however, there have been changes in nurse education, with the arrival of Project 2000, new specific measures by the Royal College of Nursing regarding standards of care in cancer nursing and the European Oncology Nursing Society's current developments for a core curriculum for post-basic cancer courses. These initiatives represent a significant move away from a biomedical model towards a humanistic approach for the nursing care of persons with cancer. However, for the present, the arguments used here attempt to explain the reasons behind the mismatch of philosophies discovered from the interview data.

To conclude, it cannot simply be implied from the interview data that there are a significant proportion of nurses who adopt a humanistic approach and subsequently explore the person with cancer's perceptions of stress. Rather, an analysis of the interview data reveals two key contrasting philosophies. Overall, there is a biomedical approach, yet within the layers of consciousness of the nurses, there also lies a humanistic approach.

Observation findings

A discussion of the key philosophy emerging from the non-participant observation of the nursing admission assessments of persons with cancer
The overall philosophy underpinning the observations is much more clear cut and conclusive than the philosophies reflected in the interview findings. It can be seen in Chapter 9 that the biomedical model represents the approach adopted by the majority of nurses during the respective nursing admission assessments. As argued in previous research findings, the cancer nurses are primarily concerned with the physiological aspects of a person's illness, to the relative exclusion of psychosocial aspects of care. Despite a humanistic approach being reflected in several key themes within the interviews, the overall philosophy of biomedicine clearly prevails

within the routine implementation of nursing admission assessments of persons with cancer.

Given the reality of nurses' everyday clinical practice, it is much more likely that the medical model represents the overriding approach. Despite being aware (albeit subconsciously in some cases) of a person's psychosocial concerns, the cancer nurses fail to acknowledge or act on these concerns. Therefore, a humanistic approach is not followed through into their routine nursing practice. Rather, the nurses rely on the familiar practices inherent within the powerful medical model (i.e. a medicalised assessment which focuses on the physiological signs and symptoms of the disease and in which information is restricted largely to the side-effects of the treatment).

The admission assessment is doctor-oriented due to the commanding role of medical forms of therapy (i.e. cytotoxic, chemotherapy, radiotherapy) to treat cancer. As argued earlier in the interview findings, this is reflected in the previous nurse education of qualified nurses. The medical emphasis provided in nurse training, prior to the advent of Project 2000 (with the exclusion of degree courses in nursing) is also reinforced in the nursing Kardex. The printed emphasis (similar to a medical assessment) on physiological aspects of a person's illness becomes translated into nursing practice during the nursing admission assessment of the person with cancer. Despite the current changes in nurse education and the growing public and professional awareness of the importance of support for persons with cancer, change is slow. As previously argued by Deeley (1979), it takes a significant period of time for attitudes to change.

Unfortunately, it may take a further period of time (i.e. after several years of successive nursing students having achieved registered general nurse status via Project 2000 courses and degree courses) before radical changes occur in the way in which cancer nurses carry out the admission assessments of persons with cancer. In addition, current qualified nurses also need ready access to post-registration courses which focus on their psychological support role and the use of specialist communication and counselling skills.

The use of methodological triangulation for the study proved invaluable, as it allowed an exploration of the differences between what cancer nurses say in one context, and what they actually do in another, clinical context. It has been possible to verify information from informants' reports of behaviour during the interviews, with actual behaviour in the everyday setting. The use of observation findings has increased the validity of the study and supports the argument that the use of a single method (e.g. the in-depth interview) often leads to a distorted and limited view of human behaviour.

The differences between reported and actual behaviour can be clearly seen regarding the psychological support role of the cancer nurse. In the interviews, all the nurses emphasised the central importance of their support role. However, this role was not in evidence in the majority of admission assessments, as there were key areas of omission in relation to a person's psychological state, coping mechanisms, communication patterns with family or significant others, perception of treatment, reaction to hospital and hospitalisation. It is interesting to note that a third of respondents in the interviews acknowledged that they required further training in psychosocial aspects of care and several respondents spoke of the constraints on them which made the implementation of their support role difficult. Both these sets of respondents have helped to explain the differences in the findings.

The old cliche, 'it is one thing to say something but quite another to actually do it', applies to the highlighted difference in findings between the two research methods. For example, in the interviews most nurses spoke of the effects of cancer on partner relationships and explored this by giving examples of individuals they had nursed. However, in the admission assessments, none of the nurses explored the communication patterns between the individual with cancer and his/her family (e.g whether the individual was able to discuss his/her worries with family or friends). It can be argued that, within the admission assessment, it is unusual and sometimes inappropriate to ask in-depth questions regarding and individual's personal life, as it may prove embarrassing for the individual concerned. However, in the observation findings, several persons with cancer revealed their concern for their partners. Also, several gave references to their concern regarding their ability to manage in the home. Hence, both explicit and implicit references were given, which directly related to partner relationships, yet these were not subsequently explored by any of the respective nurses. This clearly relates to Maguire's findings that nurses fail to clarify a person's responses, thus effectively blocking communication regarding his/her concerns.

The disparity between the findings is also apparent in relation to indicators of stress. A third of nurse respondents spoke of the importance of non-verbal cues, yet, during the admission assessments, only a minority of nurses picked up on the non-verbal cues of persons with cancer (even though the research directly observed overt signs of anxiety in the majority of individuals with cancer). This supports the earlier argument of nurses being primarily concerned with the physiological aspects of a person's illness, to the exclusion of psychosocial aspects of care (in keeping with a biomedical approach).

It is also interesting to note that, although most of the nurses explored the persons' perceptions of their illness and a third of individuals openly stated that they had cancer, only one nurse subsequently explored a person's perceptions regarding cancer. However, in the interviews, all the nurses acknowledged that the negative attitudes surrounding cancer were often an over-riding concern for persons with cancer. Part of the reason for this concern is suggested by the interview findings, as the majority of nurse respondents acknowledged that few persons actually express their negative thoughts about having cancer. Also, most nurse respondents perceived cancer as stigmatising and several admitted that health care professionals often have negative views regarding cancer. The inference is that negative views by persons with cancer are normal and, thus, are not deemed in need of exploration unless severe psychological problems develop.

The prevalence of the biomedical model in the admission assessments is clearly highlighted in the areas of omission, which relate to exploration of persons' perceptions regarding psychological aspects of their care. For example, in the interviews, half of the nurses spoke of the powerful stigmatising effects of the hospital itself. Yet, during the admission assessments, despite half of the nurses asking respective individuals with cancer about their reaction to hospitalisation, only one nurse explored the effects of the hospital itself on the person. Similarly, in the interviews nearly half of the nurses explained the stigma relating to the nature of the treatment given, yet, in the admission assessments, the majority of nurses focused on the individual's illness (in keeping with a biomedical approach). Three quarters of the nurses gave information relating to treatment, while only a third of the nurses explored persons' perceptions of the treatment itself. This relates to Maguire's findings that nurses often fail to establish how persons have been affected by the information given about treatment and by their perceptions of the treatment.

It can also be argued that, in the majority of nursing admission assessments, the nurses failed to take on board the wider psychological effects of cancer on the individual. In the interviews, half of the nurses spoke of the loss of plans for the future and gave specific examples to highlight the loss involved. Also, over half of the nurses spoke of the sense of failure and frustration experienced by individuals with cancer who were no longer able to carry out their previous roles. However, in the admission assessments, very few of the nurses explored the emotional effects of cancer when individuals with cancer outlined their main concerns. Thus, the majority of nurses maintained an emotional distance, in keeping with Maguire's findings.

This emotional distancing is also clearly evident with respect to the subject of coping. During the interviews, the majority of respondents listed a diverse range of coping patterns and also gave specific examples of individuals to substantiate their views. However, in the nursing admission assessments, only one nurse directly asked a person with cancer how he/she was coping with the illness. It appears that the humanistic approach reflected in the interviews is not actively carried through into nurses' clinical practice. Therefore, nurses being aware of psychosocial issues affecting the person with cancer is not enough to ensure that they directly explore these areas in the admission assessments. It can be argued that the nursing admission assessment forms only one aspect of nursing care, albeit a significant one. Therefore, it is possible that psychosocial aspects of care could have been explored at a later stage, although research findings reveal that this does not usually occur.

As previously argued, the reasons for this neglect of the psychosocial aspects of care stem from a lack of education in communication and counselling skills within a central humanistic framework. Education in this area would enable nurses to learn how to help persons with cancer explore their psychosocial concerns. Thus, the previous emphasis on the biomedical model in nurse education, in addition to the medicalised form of the nursing Kardex, creates the chasm between the awareness of psychosocial aspects of cancer nursing care and the actual implementation of cancer nursing care.

It is important not to underestimate the significance of situational constraints which are of current concern in the general nursing press and which were clearly vocalised by the majority of nurses in the interviews. For example, the situation of a heavy workload in proportion to inadequate numbers of qualified staff on duty leads to a perceived lack of time. When this occurs, several respondents acknowledged that acute physical needs predominate over psychological ones, as these nurses' rationalise that the latter can be addressed at a later date, whereas acute physical care needs often require immediate attention (e.g. care of people receiving platelets, or care of the person who is vomiting). This helps to explain why a biomedical model prevails in actual nursing practice.

Archival sources

A discussion of the key philosophy emerging from the archival sources
Similar to the observation findings, the overall philosophy underpinning the archival sources is well-defined, as opposed to the more amorphous nature of the philosophies present within the interview findings. The biomedical model is clearly in evidence in the nursing Kardexes analysed, as the key areas recorded were the person's perceptions of the illness, the physiological effects of the illness on the person (e.g the effects on the person's daily living activities) and practical details of the individual's social circumstances. The sparse and, hence, superficial picture gained of these areas reflects the lack of adequate space to record the individual's perceptions of the illness, treatments and reaction to hospitalisation. It also highlights the lack of specific space to record relevant psychosocial needs.

As in previous research findings (see p63), such as those of Fox and Camp (1988), the archival sources revealed that the nurses' documentation of patient care was inadequate. For example, there was routine use of the words 'anxiety' and 'adjustment' and there were inconsistencies present regarding an individual's reaction to hospitalisation. In the current era of technology and the use of computers, it is of increasing importance that nurses are able to record concise and clear information regarding psychosocial aspects of a person's care. Otherwise, recorded data will continue to focus almost exclusively on physiological aspects of care, in keeping with the current medicalisation of the nursing Kardex. This will probably result in the psychological needs of individuals with cancer remaining unmet.

As the interview findings proved, it is not sufficient for nurses to be aware of the present situation. For example, in the interviews, most of the nurses were aware of the positive aspects of the nursing process, yet none of these positive aspects were actually reflected in the completed nursing Kardexes. It is also interesting to note that the majority of respondents acknowledged that the nursing Kardex was not being used effectively in everyday clinical practice. However, this awareness *per se* is insufficient to bring about changes in the way in which data is recorded. In their initial education, nurses require appropriate training in modes of communication, and current qualified staff require appropriate post-registration training in written communication. At the same time, the nursing Kardex needs to be urgently revised to incorporate an humanistic philosophy in which the psychosocial needs, in addition to the physiological needs, are systematically explored and concisely recorded.

This leads into the next section regarding an appropriate theory base for cancer nurses to use in their clinical practice, in order to actively address the psychosocial needs of the person with cancer.

A humanistic model of care

A proposal for the humanistic model for the psychosocial care of persons with cancer

Cancer nurses require an appropriate theoretical approach, which draws on their awareness of the perceptions of stress amongst persons with cancer. The adoption of a philosophy which is totally new and, hence, alien to the cancer nurse is not being advocated here. Rather, it is proposed that use should be made of the taken-for-granted world of the cancer nurse in relation to stress and persons with cancer. This involves shaping the nurses' humanistic interpretations (often lying within their consciousness) into a coherent and explicit whole, in order to place the biomedical model within the holistic framework of the psychosocial, as well as the physiological needs of the person with cancer.

A descriptive framework, as highlighted by the nurses in the interviews and in keeping with a phenomenological approach, is proposed. A prescriptive approach, indicative of a biomedical model, is clearly inappropriate, as it has a tendency to stereotype persons, thus reducing the complexity and diversity of stress as applied to persons with cancer. It is highly unsuitable to infer the notion of a rigid, hierarchical list of nursing orders for the the cancer nurse to follow (as represented in the traditional role of the nurse as handmaiden to the doctor). It can be seen that a prescriptive framework reflects a behaviourist approach, due to its restrictive focus on the prerequisites necessary to implement a nursing model. The set criteria are generally cumbersome and confusing and, therefore, are not amenable to clinical nursing practice. In contrast, a descriptive framework, similar to a phenomenological approach, is non-judgmental. It is directly concerned with providing the appropriate context for an account of the everyday experiences of persons with cancer, in order to gain an insight regarding their world and, thus, enable nurses to explore the individual's perceptions of stress.

Cancer nurses require an appropriate theory which is matched with common-sense views, in order to improve the delivery of care. If there is too little theory, then cancer nurses have no form of reference on which to base their care, and delivery is of an *ad hoc* nature. However, if there is too much theory, so that the common-sense interpretations of the professionals using the theory are ignored, then it becomes restrictive and ultimately meaningless.

A humanistic approach can be seen to represent the core philosophy throughout this study (see Fig. 10.1). The humanistic perceptions of the cancer nurse are vividly seen (e.g. in relation to discussion of the family and the complex relationships involved; the notion of psychological helplessness regarding change in roles; the effect of cancer on future plans; the psychological effects of altered body image). Humanism relates to the practice of regarding things in their true nature and dealing with them as they are, to the freedom from prejudices and convention and to the pursuit of practical views

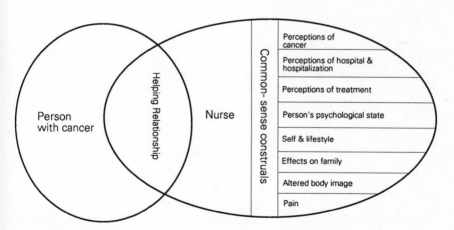

Figure 10.1: Diagrammatic representations of a humanistic model for the psychosocial care of persons with cancer

and policy. It also includes an insistence on details and the showing of life as it is without glossing over what is considered to be ugly or painful.

It is important for nurses working with persons with cancer to accept that stress is highly probable amongst persons with cancer, given the prevalent stigmatising views discussed in the study. However, by accepting this probability of stress a negative approach is not being inferred, rather the reality of the situation is being acknowledged. We are fooling ourselves if we do not work from this premise and, instead employ cognitive coping strategies ourselves to ignore its existence. Surely, a negative approach would be implied if, having acknowledged the likelihood of stress in persons with cancer, we accepted the situation *per se* and did not take any appropriate supportive action to reduce the stress as far as possible? This acceptance of the situation currently occurs in clinical practice, due to the predominance of the biomedical model.

A central theme of a humanistic approach is acknowledging stress amongst persons with cancer and subsequently exploring the roots of stress amongst individuals with cancer. In this way, a person's perceptions of cancer and its treatment can be discovered. The use of a humanistic framework would help to ensure that a systematic approach was adopted. It would also ensure that key psychosocial areas (e.g. perceptions of cancer; perceptions of hospital and hospitalisation; perceptions of treatment; person's psychological state; self and lifestyle; effects on family; altered body image; pain), raised in the interviews by nurses and highlighted in the literature, were assessed.

Information regarding a person's perceptions of stress could be used subsequently, to gain an understanding of how the person is coping with the illness and a possible insight into the reasons why the person is coping in a particular way, at a given moment in time (i.e. initially on admission to hospital and then throughout the duration of the person's stay in hospital). Advocating a humanistic method with respect to the relationship between stress and persons with cancer, does not infer the superiority of more 'realistic' forms of coping. As seen in the interview findings, individuals with cancer cope with their illness in very different ways. What may be considered by 'outsiders' as more unrealistic and inappropriate forms of coping, may be the only current avenues open to the individual concerned. For example, denial may constitute a useful form of coping for an individual who has recently been diagnosed as having a malignant illness. The use of a humanistic approach would help to further explore the probable reasons for coping in this way, and, hence, respect the individual's mode of coping, at the given moment in time.

Having carried out a systematic assessment of a person's perceptions of stress and ways of coping, the active implementation of psychosocial care should be encouraged, via the cancer nurse's support role. Thus, an open approach and appropriate specialist communication skills and non-directive counselling techniques (as highlighted in the health research literature, see Chapter 4) should be used, in order to reduce a person's stress as much as possible.

It is important for cancer nurses to continually evaluate their psychosocial care of persons with cancer, because of the constant flux regarding stress and coping amongst persons with cancer. Thus, the humanistic model of care is a dynamic process, in keeping with Lazarus' transactional model of stress and coping (1966).

Recommendations

The following recommendations arise from the discussion:
i)   – For the use of the humanistic model as an appropriate foundation for the nursing care of persons with cancer.

– To build on the nurses' common-sense knowledge and understanding of the world of the person with cancer.

– To substantiate the nurses' perceptions by reference to relevant health research, literature and psychological concepts, in order to create a sound knowledge base for nurses with regard to psychosocial aspects of care for persons with cancer.

– For the knowledge base to act as a core element in cancer care course curricula for pre/post-credential courses and degree courses for nurses and possibly other health professionals, such as medical social workers and clinical psychologists (particularly those wishing to specialise in the care of persons with cancer).

– For the described educational foundation to create a shift in emphasis away from a medical model, which accentuates the 'patient', towards a humanistic approach, which focuses on the 'person'.

ii)   – For staff support to be recognised as essential by health services management, in order to actively address the psychosocial needs of persons with cancer. That is, the management should recognise the need for adequate numbers and skill mixes of staff and the staff's need for psychological support (e.g. supportive nurse managers, use of support groups). The research project on which this book is based is one way of addressing the psychosocial care of persons with cancer. However, the development of further research projects which focus on support measures (both informal and formal) for staff, within the current constraints of the National Health Service, is urgently required.

This study has examined the concept of stress amongst persons with cancer, which is often taken for granted by nurses. As a result, a person's experience of stress may be ignored and may not be explored on an individual level by the nurse. Cancer nurses should reflect carefully on the concept of stress amongst persons with cancer. Failure to consider stress in the individual with cancer can result in harmful consequences. Cancer nurses must use their common-sense knowledge and everyday understanding of the world of the person with cancer to assess the person's psychosocial needs. This book lays down a useful knowledge base which enables nurses to adopt a humanistic approach for the care of persons with cancer.

Bibliography

Albrecht G L (1977). The Negotiated Diagnosis and Treatment of Occlusal Problems in Health/Illness in Medicine, Higgins P ed, *A Reader in Medical Sociology*, Rand McNally, New York.

Ainsley S (1984). Sexuality and the Cancer Sufferer, *Nurs Mirror*, **159**, 10, 38–40.

Baum M and Jones E M (1979). Counselling removes patient's fears, *Nurs Mirror*, **148**, 10, 38–40.

Baxley K *et al* (1984). Alopecia: Effect on cancer patient's body image, *Cancer Nurs*, December, 499–503.

Benner P and Wrubel J (1989). *The Primacy of Caring — Stress and Coping in Health and Illness*, Addison Wesley, California.

Blackmore C (1988a). The impact of orchidectomy upon the sexuality of the man with testicular cancer, *Cancer Nurs*, **11**, 1, 33—40.

Blackmore C (1988b). Body Image — the Oncology Perspective, Salter M ed, *Altered Body Image, the Nurse's Role*, John Wiley, Chichester.

Bond S (1978). Processes of Communication about Cancer in a Radiotherapy Department, *Unpublished thesis*, University of Edinburgh.

Bond S (1982). Communication in Cancer Nursing, Cahoon M ed, *Recent Advances in Cancer Nursing*, Churchill Livingstone, London, pp3–31.

Bonica (1990). *The Management of Pain*, Lea and Felsiger, Pennsylvania

Bridge W and MacLeod Clark J (1981). *Communication in Nursing Care*, HM and M, London.

Buckalew P G (1982). A nurse clinician's experiences and anxiety during chemotherapy, *Cancer Nurs*, **5**, 6, 435–440.

Bullough B (1981). Nurses as teachers and support persons, *Cancer Nurs*, **4**, 3, 221–225.

Burish T and Carey M (1986). Conditioned aversive responses in cancer chemotherapy patients: Theoretical and developmental analysis, *J Clinical Psychol*, **54**, 5, 593–600.

Camp F (1989). Sexuality and the cancer patient; The nurse's role, *Cancer Nurs*, **12**, 1 46–53.

Camp L D (1988). A comparison of nurses' recorded assessments of pain with perceptions of pain as described by cancer patients, *Cancer Nurs*, **11**, 4, 237–243.

Chapman C (1979). Psychologic and Behavioural Aspects of Cancer Pain, Bonica J and Ventafridda V eds, *Advances in Pain and Research Therapy*, Volume 2, International Symposium on Pain of Advanced Cancer, Raven Press, New York.

Corkle R (1984) *Patient Education: Its Role in Cancer Nursing in the 80s*, Proceedings of the 3rd International Conference of Cancer Nursing, Balliere Tindall, Melbourne.

Cox T (1978). *Stress*, Macmillan, London.

Craytor J and Fass H (1982). Changing nurses' perceptions of cancer and cancer care, *Cancer Nurs*, February, 43–49.

Davitz Jr and Davitz L L (1981). Inferences of patients' pain and psychological distress, *Studies of Nursing Behaviours*, Springer Verlag, New York.

Deeley T (1979). *Attitudes to Cancer*, SPCK, London.

Derogatis L R and Kourtesis S M (1981). An approach to evaluation of sexual problems of the cancer patient, *CA-A Cancer J Clinicians*, **31**, 4, 46–50.

Devlen J (1984). Psychological Aspects of Hodgkin's Disease and Non-Hodgkin's Lymphoma, *Unpublished thesis*, University of Manchester.

Dimbleby R and Burton G (1985). *More Than — An Introduction to Communication*, Metheun, London.

Dingwall R (1976). *Aspects of Illness*, Martin Roberston, London.

Doyal L and Epstein S (1983). *Cancer in Britain: The Politics of Prevention*, Pluto Press, London.

Elkind A (1982). Nurses' views about cancer, *J Adv Nurs*, **7**, 43–50.

Fallowfield L (1988). Psychological Complications of Malignant Disease, Kaye S and Rankin E eds, Medical complications of malignant disease, *Balliere's Clinical Oncology International Practice and Research, July 1988*, **2**, 2, 461–478.

Fredette S and Beattie H (1986). Living with cancer — A patient education programme, *Cancer Nurs*, **9**, 6, 308–316.

Freud S (1924). *Collected Papers 2, 3, 4*, Hogarth Press and Institute Psychoanalysis, London.

Friedenbergs I *et al* (1980). Assessment and treatment of psychosocial problems of the cancer patient: A case study. *Cancer Nurs*, **3**, 111–119.

Friedson (1968). Perceptions of illness-role of patient, in Mechanic D (ed), *Medical sociology: A selective view*, Free Press, New York.

Glaser B and Strauss A (1967). *The Discovery of Grounded Theory: Strategies for Qualitative Research*, Aldine Press, New York.

Glass D C and Singer J E (1972). *Urban Stress: Experiment on Noise and Social Stressors*, RP, New York.

Glover J (1985). *Human Sexuality in Nursing Care*, Croom Helm, London

Goffman I (1963). *Stigma: Notes on the Management of Spoiled Identity*, Penguin, London.

Goffman I (1967). *Asylums: Essays on the Social Situation of Mental Patients and Other Inmates*, Penguin, London.

Goldberg R J and Cullen L O (1986). Depression in geriatric cancer patients: A guide to assessment and treatment, *Hospice J*, **2**, 2, 79–80.

Golden J S (1983). Sex and cancer, *Danish Medical Bull 30: Supplement 2*, 4–6

Hayward J (1975). *Information — A Prescription Against Pain*, RCN Series 2 No 5, London

Henry I C (1986) Concepts of the Nature of Persons Amongst Children and Adolescents, *Unpublished thesis*, University of Leeds.

Herzlich C (1973). *Health and Illness*, Academic Press, London.

Hitch P and Murgatroyd J (1983). Professional communications in cancer care: A Delphi survey of hospital nurses, *J Adv Nurs*, **8**, 413–422.

Hoffman N (1977). *A New World of Health*, McGraw-Hill, New York.

Hogan R (1980). *Human Sexuality: A Nursing Perspective*, Appleton Century Crofts, New York.

Holmes S (1985). Pursuits of Happiness, *Nurs Mirror*, **161**, 13, 438.

Holmes T and Rahe R (1967). The social readjustment and rating scale, *J Psych Res*, **11**, 213–218.

Huskinsson E C (1979). Visual analogue scales, Bonica J and Ventafridda V eds, *Advances in Pain and Research Therapy*, Volume 2, International Symposium on Pain of Advanced Cancer, Raven Press, New York.

Izsak F and Medalie J (1971). Comprehensive follow-up of carcinoma patients, *J Chronic Disease*, **24**, 179–191.

Jamison K R, Wellisch D K and Pasnau R O (1978). Psychosocial aspects of mastectomy. The woman's perspective, *Amer J Psych*, **135**, 4, 432–436.

Johnson J (1980). A Patient's Structured Educational Programme to Help People Learn to Live with Cancer, Tiffany R ed, *Cancer Nursing Update*, Proceedings of 2nd International Cancer Nursing Conference, Balliere Tindall, London.

Johnson P (1988). Principles of Cancer Education, Tiffany R and Webb P (eds), *Oncology for Nurses and Health Care Professionals* (2 edn), Harper & Row, London.

Johnston M (1982). Recognition of patients' worries by nurses and by other patients, *Brit J Counsell Psychol*, **21**, 255–261.

Jones E (1984). A Comparative Study of the Perceptions of Young Male Patients and Nurses about Testicular Cancer, its Treatment and Prognosis, *Unpublished thesis*, Univ of Edinburgh.

Kendrick K (1991). Consideration of Personhood in Nursing Research: An Ethical Perspective, Soothill K, Henry C and Kendrick K (eds), *Themes and Perspectives in Nursing*, Harper Collins, London.

Kent G and Dalgleish M (1983). *Psychology and Medical Care*, Van Nostrand Reinholt, New York.

Kubler Ross E (1969). *On Death and Dying*, Macmillan, New York.

Lazarus R (1966). *Psychological Stress and the Coping Process*, McGraw-Hill, New York.

Lazarus R (1976). *Patterns of Adjustment* (3rd edn), McGraw-Hill, New York.

Lazarus R (1978). Stress-related transactions between person and environment, In Pervin L A and Lewis M (eds), *Perspectives in International Psychology*, Plenen Press, New York, pp287.

Lazarus R (1981). Cognitive Style, Stress Perception and Coping, In Kutashi I and Schlesinger L (eds), *Handbook on Stress and Anxiety*, Jossey Bass, New York.

Lazarus R (1984). *Stress, Appraisal and Coping*, Springer Press, New York.

Lion E M (1982). *Human Sexuality in Nursing Process*, John Wiley, New York.

Long B (1976). *Doctors Talking to Patients: A Study of Verbal Behaviour of GPs Consulting in Their Surgeries*, HMSO, London.

MacLeod Clark J (1981). Communicating with Cancer Patients: Communication of Evasion, In Tiffany R (ed), *Cancer Nursing Update*, Balliere Tindall, London.

MacLeod Clark J and Sims S (1988). Communication with Patients and Relatives, In Tiffany R and Webb P (eds), *Oncology for Nurses and Health Care Professionals* (2 edn), Harper and Row, London.

Maguire P (1978). The Psychological Effects of Cancer, Tiffany R ed, *Oncology for Nurses and Health Care Professionals*, (1 edn), Harper and Row, London.

Maguire P *et al* (1980). Planning a Caring Programme, *Nurs Mirror,* January, 35–37.

Maguire P (1985a). The psychological impact of cancer, *Brit J Hospital Med,* August, 100–193.

Maguire P (1985b). Barriers to psychological care of the dying, *B M J,* **291**, 1711–1713.

Maguire P (1985c). Psychological morbidity associated with cancer and cancer treatment, *Clinics Oncol,* **4**, 3, 559–575.

Mansfield (1976). *Op cit, Fit for the Future,* HMSO (1976), 6684.

Maslow A (1957). *Motivation and Personality (2 edn),* Harper and Row, New York.

McCaffrey M (1983). *Nursing the Patient in Pain (2 edn),* Harper and Row, New York.

McCaffrey M (1985). Perspectives in Pain, In Copp L (ed), *Recent Advances in Nursing 11,* Churchill Livingstone, London.

Mechanic D (1968). *Medical Sociology,* Macmillan, London.

Melzack R (1983). *Pain Measurement and Assessment,* Raven Press, New York.

Melzack R and Wall P (1982). *The Challenge of Pain,* Penguin, Harmondsworth.

Menzies I E (1960). A case study of the functioning of social systems as a defence against anxiety: A report on a study of the nursing service of a general hospital, *Human Relations,* **13**, 95–121.

Merskey H and Spear F G (1967). *Pain: Psychyologic and Psychiatrice Aspects,* Bailliere, Tindall and Cassel, London.

Mishel M *et al* (1984). Predictors of psychosocial adjustment in patients newly diagnosed with gynaecological cancer, *Cancer Nurs,* **7**, 4, 291–299.

Mohrer D, Arthur A Z and Pater J L (1984). Anticipatory nausea and/or vomiting, *Cancer Treatment Rev,* **11**, 257–264.

Moorey S (1988). The Psychological Impact of Cancer, In Tiffany R, Webb P (eds) *Oncology for Nurses and Health Care Professionals, (2 edn),* Harper and Row, London.

Morris T, Buckley M and Blake S M (1986). Defining Psychological Responses to a Diagnosis of Cancer, In Watson M and Morris T eds, *Psychological Aspects of Cancer,* Pergamon Press, Oxford.

Morris, T, Greer, S and Pettingale K (1981). Patterns of expressions of anger and their psychological correlates in women with breast cancer, *J Psychosom Res,* **25**, 2, 111–117.

Morrow G R *et al* (1978). A new scale for assessing patients' psychosocial adjustment to medical illness, *Psycholog Med,* **8**, 605–610.

Nichols K A (1984). Psychological care by nurses, Essential developments for the general hospital, *Brit J Med Phys,* **58**, 231–240.

Northouse L (1981). Living with Cancer, *Amer J Nurs,* **5**, 960–962.

Osborn B (1968). *Foundations of Health Science,* Allyn and Bacon, Boston.

Parker J (1981). *Cancer passage: Continuity and discontinuity in terminal illness,* Unpub doctoral dissertation, Monash Univ, Australia.

Parker J (1985). Cancer Passage — The Change Process in Leukaemia, In King K (ed), *Long Term Care, Recent Advances in Nursing,* Churchill Livingstone, London, pp96–119.

Parsons T (1951). *The Social System,* Free Press, London.

Pearson A (1987). *Primary Nursing: Nursing in the Burford and Oxford Nursing Development Units,* John Wiley, Chichester.

Peters-Golden H (1982). Breast cancer: Varied perceptions of social support in the illness experience, *Social Sci Med,* **16**, 483–491.

Poletti R (1984). Helping people to cope with stress, *Nurs Times,* **80**, 13, 47–49.

Pugsley R and Pardoe J (1988). The Sociological Impact of Cancer, In Tiffany R and Webb P (eds), *Oncology for Nurses and Health Care Professionals* (2 edn), Volume 2, Care and Support, Harper Row, London.

Raiman J (1986). The London Hospital Pain Chart, In Wilson Barnett J and Raiman J (eds), *Nursing Issues and Research in Terminal Care,* John Wiley, Chichester.

Raiman J (1988). Pain and its Management, In Wilson Barnett J and Raiman J (eds), *Nursing Issues and Research in Terminal Care — Development in Nursing Research,* Volume 6, John Wiley, Chichester.

Rogers C (1973). *On Becoming a Person,* Constable, London.

Rowat K (1985). Chronic Pain, In King K (ed), *Long Term Care, Recent Advances in Nursing,* Churchill Livingstone, London.

Rutherford D (1988). Assessing psychosocial needs of women experiencing lumpectomy – challenge for research, *Cancer Nurs,* **1**, 4, 244–250.

Salter M (1988). Normal and Altered Body Image, In Salter M (ed), *Altered Body Image: The Nurse's Role,* John Wiley, Chichester.

Saunders C (1984) *The Management of Terminal Malignant Disease,* (2 edn), Edward Arnold, London.

Seligman H (1975). *Helplessness on Depression, Development and Death,* W H Freeman/Scribner, New York.

Selye H (1957). *The Stress of Life,* McGraw-Hill, New York.

Silberfarb P M (1978). Psychiatric themes in the rehabilitation of mastectomy patients, *Intnl J Psychol Med,* **8**, 2, 159–167.

Smith D (1989). Sexual rehabilitation of the cancer patient, *Cancer Nurs,* **12**, 1, 10–15

Sofaer B (1984). *Pain: A Handbook for Nurses,* Harper and Row, London.

Sontag I (1979). *Illness as a Metaphor,* Harper and Row, London.

Strauss A (1978). *Negotiation: Varieties, Contexts, Processes and Social Order,* Jossey Bass, New York.

Sternbach R (1978). Clinical Aspects of Pain, In Sternbach R (ed), *Psychology of Pain,* Raven Press, New York, pp241–265.

Stockwell F (1980). *The Unpopular Patient,* RCN Research Project Series 1, No 2, London.

Stromberg M and Wright P (1984). Ambulatory cancer patients' perceptions of the physical and psychosocial changes in their lives since the diagnosis of cancer, *Cancer Nurs,* **17**, 2, 117–131.

Tait A *et al* (1982). Improving communication skills, *Nurs Times,* **78**, 51 2181–2184.

Tait A (1988). Whole or Partial Breast Loss: The Threat to Womanhood, In Salter M (ed), *Altered Body Image: The Nurse's Role,* John Wiley, Chichester.

Tuckett D (1976). *An Introduction to Medical Sociology,* Tavistock, London.

Turner C (1985). Patient Education, *Senior Nurse,* **12**, 2, 10–12.

Vachon M L S *et al* (1978). Measurement and management of stress in health professionals working with advanced cancer patients, *Death Education*, **1**, 365–375.

Van Eschenbach A C and Shover L R (1984). Sexual Rehabilitation of Cancer Patients, In Gunn A E (ed), *Cancer Rehabilitation*, Raven Press, New York, pp155–173.

Wassner A (1982). The impact of mutilating surgery or trauma on body image, *Intnl Nurs Rev*, **29**, 86–90.

Waugh L (1988). Psychological aspects of cancer pain, *Profess Nurse*, September, 504–506.

Webb C (1985). *Sexuality, Nursing and Health*, John Wiley, Chichester.

Webb P (1988). Teaching Patients and Relatives, In Tiffany R and Webb P (eds), *Oncology for Nurses and Health Care Professionals* (2 edn), Harper and Row, London.

Weisman A D (1979). *Coping with Cancer*, McGraw-Hill, New York.

Welch McCaffrey D (1984). Oncology nurses as cancer patients: An investigative questionnaire, *Oncol Nurs Forum*, **11**, 2, 48–50.

Welch McCaffrey D (1985). Cancer, anxiety and quality of life, *Cancer Nurs*, **8**, 3, 151–158.

Whelan J (1984). Oncology Nurses' attitudes toward cancer treatment and survival, *Cancer Nurs*, **7**, 5, 375–383.

Witts P (1992). Patient advocacy in nursing, In Soothill K, Henry C and Kendrick K (eds), *Themes and Perspectives in Nursing*, Harper Collins, London.

Wright K And Dyck S (1984). Expressed concerns of adult cancer patients' family members, *Cancer Nurs*, **7**, 5, 371–375.

Young L and Longman A (1983). Quality of life and persons with melanoma: A pilot study, *Cancer Nurs*, **6**, 3, 219–225.

Zborowski M (1969). *People in Pain*, Jossey Bass, San Fransisco.

Zola I K (1966). Culture and symptoms: An analysis of patients' presenting complaints, *Amer Sociol Rev*, **XXXI**, 615.#

Index